Epilepsy Surgery
A Guide For Patients and Families

RUBEN KUZNIECKY, M.D.

NYU Langone Comprehensive Epilepsy Center

Professor of Neurology

New York Universal Medical Center

New York

With contributions by:

Werner Doyle, M.D., Associate Professor of Neurosurgery at New York University

Alyson Silverberg, N.P.

DEDICATION

Dedicated to my mother, Sara, who at 87 years is as restless, fearless, and creative as a child.

TABLE OF CONTENTS

ACKNOWLEDGMENTS

This idea of this book and some of its writings started 5 years ago, but it was not until this past year that I finally got the impetus to put all of it together. It was in some way hastened by the experience of a few patients who, hesitating whether to have surgery or not, devoted many hours on the phone and in meetings with a number of health care professionals, families, and friends discussing their options. It became clear to me that providing written information to patients before epilepsy surgery would be enormously beneficial to both patients and doctors.

I am thankful to a lot of people who assisted with this project. Many people contributed with ideas and suggestions. I am particularly indebted to Foram Mehta, who I had the privilege to care for before and after her epilepsy surgery. Foram contributed to the book with her personal story, edits, and with many suggestions. I am also indebted to Alyson Silverberg. Alyson, who is a nurse practitioner at NYU, has been at the forefront of epilepsy surgery care for over 20 years. She reviewed and edited all of the nursing care issues discussed in this book. Special thanks to my surgical colleagues, Drs. Werner Doyle and Howard Weiner, awesome neurosurgeons and caring doctors. They graciously reviewed and provided many suggestions for the surgical chapters. I extend a special thanks to Isabel De Obaldia, a talented Panamanian artist, for lending us the use of her artwork for the book's cover.

I am also thankful to Nako Ishii, Kim Parker, Mary Micelli, Steve Pacia, Chad Carlson, Blanca Vazquez, Patricia Dugan, and many other members of our team who were helpful by providing ideas and material for this book. Thanks also to the patients who contributed to Chapter 9 with their perspective, ideas, and comments. Particular thanks also to my son Joel Kuzniecky, whose command of the King's English made my job easier.
Special love and appreciation to my wife and children. I am guilty for spending less time with my wife Yvonne and my kids while writing this book. I hope they will forgive me.

Finally, I am deeply thankful to our patients and their families. Their enormous bravery facing epilepsy surgery is inspiring and humbling. I continue to learn every day from their experiences, successes, and failures.

Letter From a Patient Who Received Epilepsy Surgery

Date: 10/2/2004

Dear Dr. Kuzniecky:

I received your letter concerning your move to New York. I regret that I will be losing you as my doctor, but am glad for your advancement in the medical service.
I have not had a seizure since my surgery on April 22, 2003. Prior to surgery the seizures were frequent and had been a part of my life since 1967 as a PhD student at Texas A&M University. After completing my degree in 1969, I took a job at the University of Georgia, but quit after 3 years when the seizures became debilitating, moved my family back home to Prattville, began farming, and retired here. My only regret is that I did not receive help other than medication many years earlier.

INTRODUCTION

If you are reading this book, it is likely that you have a diagnosis of epilepsy or you know someone in your family or a friend who has epilepsy. It is also likely that you or that person is considering surgical intervention to treat this condition because medications or other treatments are not helping. Even though you may have knowledge and experience about epilepsy, I would like to start this book with some basic concepts.

Epilepsy is not a disease or a diagnosis. To say that a person has epilepsy has no specific meaning, and it should not be considered a final diagnosis. While it may give a general indication of the nature of a problem, the term is so unspecific as to be almost meaningless in many ways. "Epilepsy" includes many conditions that can manifest in many ways. Epilepsy can result from an injury to the brain, a brain infection, a brain tumor, inflammation, or the interplay of abnormal genes that can cause epilepsy with or without other symptoms. A seizure is simply a manifestation of abnormal neuronal function (that is, neurons are firing abnormally due to different reasons; see Chapter 1). In the 21st century, we must be more specific about the type of epilepsy and the cause because the treatment will be different.

The brain is the most beautiful and complex organ in humans and in animals. Thus, is very sensitive to minor changes in function. If something goes wrong, the problem will manifest itself in abnormal functioning in various systems, such as problems with vision, hearing, language, memory, behavior, and the like. In simpler terms, abnormal brain function can be exposed by either a loss of function or an excess of activity due mostly to an imbalance between systems. As we know, seizures or epilepsy can also arise from too much abnormal activity in a brain region or through the entire brain.

Historical Background

In the earliest writings, the "sacred disease" of epilepsy was though to be caused by evil spirits or punishment by the gods. The word *epilepsy* is derived from the Greek verb *epilamvanein*, which means "to be seized," and it is associated with possession by evil spirits. The Mesopotamian and Egyptian civilizations knew of the disease for centuries. The Bible alludes to epilepsy. The Greek physicians of Hippocrates's school mentioned epilepsy as the sacred disease, despite the fact that the Greeks rejected the idea that epilepsy was a form of punishment inflicted by the gods. On the contrary, they believed that something in the brain was its cause. Even though they attempted to refute its connection to the supernatural, the treatment of epilepsy remained attached to charlatans, superstition, and magic powers for many centuries.

In the Middle Ages, fear of epilepsy and seizures became radicalized. People with epilepsy were accused of possession by devils and were targeted for death, which wrought much destruction on many people, particularly women who were often accused of witchcraft. If patients continued to have seizures despite exorcism, they were frequently put to death. Even at the end of the 19th century, it was possible for a reputable medical practitioner specializing in the treatment of epilepsy to advocate in a lecture in New York that various forms of mutilation were appropriate for the treatment of epilepsy—including castration because convulsions were believed to originate in the testes, and masturbation was believed to exacerbate epileptic seizures.

The modern view of epilepsy originated with John Hughlings Jackson (1835–1911), an Englishman physician born in Green Hammerton near Yorkshire, England. At the age of 27, Jackson was appointed as assistant physician to the National Hospital for the Relief and Cure of the Paralyzed and Epileptic (now the National Hospital for Neurology and Neurosurgery), Queen Square, London. As in many cases in medicine, Jackson had a close but unfortunate relationship with epilepsy—his wife Elizabeth Dade Jackson developed motor seizures following a stroke at a young age. During the attacks, her hand began jerking, then her leg, then her face. This type of epilepsy, with its typical march of symptoms, became known as Jacksonian epilepsy. Since Jackson was puzzled by brain function, he used his observations to develop a view of neurology that related where functions were located in the brain. In 1873, Jackson presented his classic definition of epileptic seizures as "occasional sudden excessive, rapid, and local discharges of gray matter." This view established focal seizures as being truly epileptic in origin.

The combination of scientific research and clinical findings enabled

Jackson's ideas to be confirmed by other scientists performing experiments in animals. As a result, the first step of the modern era of epilepsy treatment began.

Epilepsy Surgery

Using this incredible skill for brain localization and using the patient's complaints as a guide to the site of the seizure focus, in 1879, a neurosurgeon in Glasgow, William Macewen (1848–1924), correctly localized a brain tumor and undertook surgery to cure epilepsy based only on the symptoms. Following tumor removal, the patient survived and became seizure-free. Almost simultaneously, in London, H. Jackson convinced a young neurosurgeon named Victor Horsley (1857–1916) to operate on a young man who had frequent seizures due to a head injury caused by being kicked in the head by a horse. This case, in addition to a few others, represents the origin of neurosurgery for the treatment of epilepsy. Although these early cases were successful, establishing the principle of seizure control by surgical removal of the "seizure focus," the success of surgery for epilepsy was poor, and eventually operative treatment fell into disuse.

The Modern Era

In the early 1930s, the American neurosurgeon Wilder Penfield founded the Montreal Neurologic Institute at McGill University in Montreal with a gift from the Rockefeller Foundation. He became the lead figure in furthering the development of the surgical treatment for epilepsy and the localization of brain function. In common with Jackson, his extensive writings, coupled with a clear, detailed, and objective skills in observation, provided a wealth of information that remains important to this day. In 1929, Hans Berger, a German psychiatrist, published the technique of electroencephalogram (EEG) and showed for the first time that electrical activity of the brain could be recorded. Although Berger was disappointed that the EEG was of limited use in psychiatric patients, he showed that abnormal waves could be recorded in patients with seizures. Soon after his findings were confirmed, many centers around the world began using the EEG to study and treat patients with seizures. This was a very exciting time in neurology since, for the first time ever, physicians had a real test that could be used not only to find the area in the brain that caused seizures but also to separate different seizure types. In 1934, in Boston, Dr. Frederick Gibbs showed the spike-and-wave EEG pattern of "petite mal" for the first time, and, a few years later, Dr. Herbert Jasper worked with Wilder Penfield in Montreal to use the EEG to help in the surgical treatment of certain epilepsies. Over the next 30 years, the study of epilepsy was dominated by the technical development and understanding of the information obtained from the EEG. During this period, surgery as a treatment of epilepsy also gained considerable ground.

Epilepsy Surgery in the 21st Century

As we begin the 21st century, our treatment of epilepsy using surgical techniques has improved dramatically. We can record video-EEG as well as ambulatory EEG in patients with epilepsy for diagnosis, treatment, and surgical localization. We have many new diagnostic tests, such as modern imaging techniques like magnetic resonance imaging (MRI) and positron emission tomography (PET), sophisticated EEG/magnetoencephalogram (MEG) machines, and many other tests. Genetic testing in epilepsy is a reality now, and the number of genes found to be involved in epilepsy grows every day. Our ability to do invasive EEG is expanding, as the hardware and software are now able to record a growing number of electrodes. This new testing can help us better define who is a good candidate and who may not be a good candidate for surgery.

On the treatment aspect, we now have both responsive nerve stimulation (RNS) and MRI laser-guided treatment. Both these techniques have opened new venues for treatment and have expanded the number of candidates. The treatment of seizures and epilepsy is likely to change even more in the years to come. Robots and modeling software will be introduced in the surgical treatment in the near future. Other noninvasive surgical techniques, such as brain ultrasound treatment, local drug delivery pumps, brain wafers with anti-seizure compounds, and nano-particle drug delivery or ablation, are all possible strategies to be developed in the very near future. We hope to see them to fruition soon.

CHAPTER ONE
YOUR BRAIN AND EPILEPSY

- The brain consists of different structures and regions that control a different variety of functions.
- During a seizure, large groups of neurons are out of control. They fire excessively, and they synchronize their firing with one another.
- The term "epilepsy" is used to describe a condition in which an individual has a tendency for repeated, unprovoked seizures.
- Focal seizures originate in a discrete area in the brain. That is, the abnormal firing of neurons begins and usually stays restricted to one brain region.

The Brain: Anatomy and Function

Epilepsy and seizures originate in the brain—the mass of gelatinous material that rests inside the skull and provides us with the ability to think, speak, move, and sense, along with a variety of other functions. Just as different areas of the brain control different functions, symptoms of seizures that arise in specific regions often reflect the functions of that area. The right half of the brain controls the left side of the body, and the left half of the brain controls the right side of the body. Thus, for example, if a seizure begins in the right side of the brain, specifically in the area that controls the thumb, then the seizure may manifest itself with jerking of the left thumb or hand.

The upper brain, or *cerebrum*, is divided into left and right halves called *cerebral hemispheres*, which are connected by a bundle of nerve fibers called the *corpus callosum*. Each cerebral hemisphere contains four lobes: frontal, parietal, occipital, and temporal (Fig.1, pg. 9). Each lobe contains many different regions that control a variety of functions.

For example, in almost all right-handed individuals, the area that controls speech lies in the left frontal lobe, and the area that controls understanding of spoken and written language lies in the left temporal lobe. The lower part of the brain contains the spinal cord as well as the brainstem, which regulates sleep–wake cycles, breathing, and the heartbeat. The upper part of the brainstem contains the *thalamus*, which processes sensory information, and the *hypothalamus*, which regulates endocrine (hormone) functions through control over the pituitary gland. The lower part of the brainstem, the spinal cord, carries messages between the brain and the rest of the body.

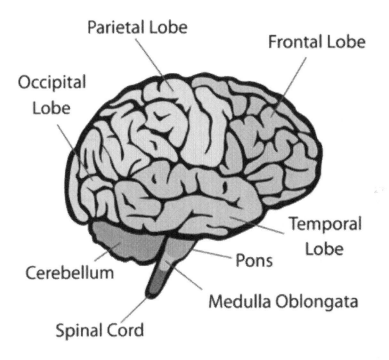

Figure 1: Brain lobes and structure.
(Athanasia Nomikou/Shutterstock)

Neurons and Neurotransmitters

Nerve cells, or *neurons*, are the building blocks of the brain. Operating like computer chips, they analyze and process complex heaps of information and then subsequently simplify and send signals through the nerve fibers. The nerve fibers act like telephone wires connecting different areas of the brain, spinal cord, muscles, and glands.

There are approximately 35 billion microscopic neurons in the brain. They are composed of three parts: the cell body, axon, and dendrites (Fig. 2, pg. 11). The cell body contains all the enzymes and chemicals that regulate the cell's metabolism and genetic information. The *axon* is the long portion of a nerve cell that resembles a wire. Axons are the "transmitting" parts of the nerve fibers and are usually surrounded by *myelin*, a fatty sheath that insulates them from and prevents cross-communication with nearby neurons. Axons also carry electrical impulses from the cell body to the end of the axon. At the end of the cell, these electrical impulses cause chemical messengers called *neurotransmitters* to be released. Neurotransmitters then cross the synapse, a tiny space between the walls of one cell's axon and the dendrite of the next nerve cell, and bind to receptors located on that dendrite. The dendrites of a neuron therefore act as "antennas," picking up on the chemical message of the neurotransmitter released from the previous neuron. There are many kinds of neurotransmitters, but each individual nerve cell produces only one major type. Some travel a long distance within the nervous system while others stay local; that is, they are produced by and released onto cells that are close to one another.

Some of the major neurotransmitters in the brain shut off or significantly decrease brain electrical activity by causing nerve cells to cease firing. These neurotransmitters are called "inhibitory" because they inhibit the activity of the cells. A neurotransmitter called gamma aminobutyric acid (GABA) is the best-known example of this type. Other neurotransmitters stimulate or increase brain electrical activity. That is, they cause or increase the firing of nerve cells. These are aptly described as "excitatory." Glutamate is one example of this type or neurotransmitter.

NEURON

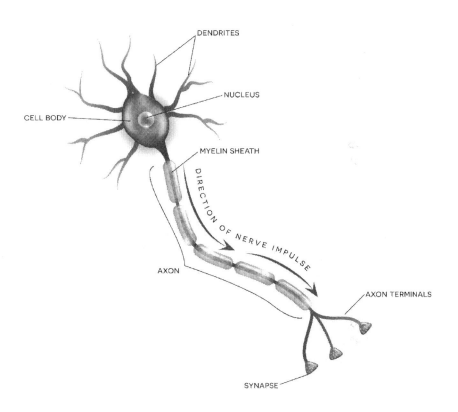

Figure 2: Neuron structure.
(Tefi/Shutterstock)

How and Why Does a Seizure Happen?

During periods of normal brain activity, neurons fire electrical impulses that influence other neurons to fire as well. The overall activity appears seemingly chaotic and arbitrary, but nonetheless results in normal functioning. In contrast to the "organized chaos" of normal brain activity, there is pure chaos during a seizure as large groups of neurons fire excessively and out of control, synchronizing their firing with one another. According to one theory, seizures are caused by an imbalance between excitatory and inhibitory neurotransmitters. If the inhibitory neurotransmitters in your brain are not active enough, or if the excitatory ones are too active, one is more likely to have seizures. Often, this "electrical storm within the brain" starts in a small, local area and gradually spreads to neighboring normal-behaving regions, causing them to act in an abnormal manner.

The spread of irregular electrical activity disrupts brain function and results in the abnormal behavior usually witnessed during a seizure. It is possible that once a seizure begins in a small group of neurons, surrounding cells are able to contain the electrical storm thus terminating the seizures. This may be deficient in some people and ends in a full-blown seizure.

What Happens Next
When a Seizure Starts and Spreads Through the Body?

A seizure may manifest itself in a multitude of ways. Seizures may cause loss of consciousness, shaking of the extremities, and other abnormal movements. Stiffness, staring spells, changes in sight or smell, hallucinations, and/or feelings of fear or déjà vu are also common. In the majority of patients, seizures generally contain themselves and end without outside intervention. In some rare cases, however, medication is needed to actively stop the seizure.

Seizure Types

Partial Seizures

A variety of seizure types exist depending on where the abnormal neuronal activity originates, the number of affected regions, and the degree to which the activity spreads. The first main category is "focal seizures." Focal seizures originate in a discrete focus in the brain. That is, the abnormal firing of neurons starts and stays restricted to one brain region. The term "partial" is used synonymously with "focal" to describe these types of seizures.

Generalized Seizures

The second category of seizures is "generalized seizures." Generalized seizures are quite different from focal (partial) seizures in that the abnormal firing seems to occur throughout the brain all at once. Research shows that, during generalized seizures, the entire brain may fire at once. However, it is possible that generalized seizures may start in one or multiple areas and spread over the brain so quickly that it is often impossible (using current methods) to detect where the first electrical discharge began.

Partial Seizures with Secondary Generalization

The last category of seizures—focal (or partial) seizures with secondary generalization—begins with a focal seizure. However, the overall state of the brain is such that the tissue surrounding the seizure focus is relatively susceptible to being too excitable and, under certain conditions, can be "recruited" to join in with the seizure focus. In this situation, the seizure focus begins to grow rapidly and spread, and it can rather quickly take over the entire brain, resulting in a generalized seizure.

Classification of the Epilepsies

Although a seizure should be thought of as a single event, the term "epilepsy" is used to describe a condition in which an individual has a tendency for repeated, unprovoked seizures. This definition implies that a person who has had only one seizure does not have epilepsy. In fact, experiencing even two or three seizures does not mean a person has epilepsy as long as the cause for the seizures can be fixed and there is no "tendency" or high likelihood for recurrences. On the other hand, in some people, one seizure may be enough to define them as having epilepsy if the likelihood of further seizures is high or tests show abnormal brain waves. In 2015, the International League Against Epilepsy (ILAE) proposed a new definition of epilepsy that includes those patients with a single seizure but with a high likelihood of further events in the future.

A person experiencing chronic seizures is usually determined to have one type of epilepsy or an epilepsy syndrome. Epilepsy is a common medical condition affecting about 2 percent of the world's population. It afflicts all age groups and appears in many varieties and forms. One individual with epilepsy may have only one type of seizure. However, another individual may have many different kinds of seizures, each of which may result in a different set of symptoms. In addition to the categories of "focal (partial)" and "generalized," which describe the origin and scope of seizures, there are additional categories that define the cause for epilepsy. These divisions, described here, are known as *idiopathic*, *symptomatic*, and *cryptogenic*.

Idiopathic Epilepsy
Idiopathic epilepsy is of unknown cause, but it is often determined to be, or thought to be, genetic. An example of this type is the syndrome of *autosomal dominant nocturnal frontal lobe epilepsy*. This epilepsy syndrome had no initial identified cause but was recognized to occur in families. Eventually, it led to the identification of a specific gene for a particular chemical receptor that caused the syndrome. Most generalized epilepsy cases are idiopathic, but more and more are being recognized as being genetic in origin. In fact, there is a case to make for calling these epilepsies *genetic generalized epilepsies* (GGE).

Symptomatic Epilepsy
Symptomatic epilepsy cases have a cause that it is usually nongenetic. The causes for such epilepsy cases are usually physical disruptions to the brain. They include head injuries, scar tissue, congenital malformations, strokes, meningitis, tumors, and bleeding. However, we know that, for example, many brain malformations causing epilepsy are genetically based. Therefore, all epilepsies, even those that are caused by physical disruption, may have a genetic background to them.

Cryptogenic Epilepsy
Cryptogenic epilepsy cases refer to those without sufficient information to determine whether they are symptomatic or idiopathic. In most of these cases, a cause is suspected but cannot be identified. For example, doctors may believe that a scar or brain abnormality is present but too small to discover with present technologies and tools. Sometimes, a patient can be classified as having cryptogenic epilepsy, but during surgery we may find a small tumor or scar tissue that was not seen on MRI.

Treatment of Epilepsy

Antiepileptic Drugs

Antiepileptic drugs (AEDs) are the principal therapy for epilepsy. These drugs attempt to decrease through a variety of mechanisms the number of seizures that an individual experiences. For example, an AED might attempt to increase the activity of inhibitory neurotransmitters, which prevent nerve cells from firing, or reduce the activity of excitatory neurotransmitters, which promote nerve cell firing. While AEDs do not cure epilepsy, they do control seizures in most people. About 65 percent of patients enjoy seizure-free lives with few medications and side effects.

Medically Intractable Epilepsy and Surgery

While most patients treated with AEDs are able to fully control their seizures, about 30–35 percent of individuals with epilepsy are not helped by medication. Patients like these are said to have "medically refractory" or "intractable" epilepsy. It is for these individuals, those who suffer with recurrent, disabling seizures, that epilepsy surgery may be considered a viable option. If the focal origin of these patients' epilepsy can be located, and the brain tissue causing it can be safely removed without impairing vital functions, surgery may result in the complete disappearance or drastic reduction of seizures. The next chapter will discuss the criteria that must be met for a person to be considered a candidate for epilepsy surgery.

CHAPTER TWO
EPILEPSY: WHO IS A SURGERY CANDIDATE?

- Patients undergoing epilepsy surgery range from infants to adults who have "intractable" or "medically refractory" epilepsy.
- Epilepsy surgery is performed on patients whose seizures have remained uncontrolled despite adequate medical treatment.
- Partial seizures are the most common type of epilepsy treated with surgery because they begin in a defined brain region.
- Epilepsy surgery can be especially beneficial to patients who have seizures associated with brain abnormalities, such as tumors, malformations, strokes, etc.

Surgery has been utilized as a treatment option for patients with epilepsy for more than a century. Its use has dramatically increased since the 1980s, rightfully reflecting its effectiveness as an alternative to seizure medications. This is largely due to advances in medical technology and patient care. However, for a variety of reasons, many physicians and patients still remain hesitant when considering surgery as an option.

According to a recent study, there may be more than 250,000 patients with epilepsy who could benefit from surgery in the United States alone, but less than 2,500 surgical procedures are performed each year in the United States. It is also estimated that between 50 and 75 percent of good surgical candidates can become seizure-free and lead relatively normal lives after surgical intervention. With state-of-the-art technology now available, patients can undergo both safe and minimally invasive procedures that will aid them in achieving the highest possible quality of life. This chapter will discuss the benefits of considering surgery and the specific criteria individuals must meet in order to be considered as viable candidates.

Medically Intractable (Refractory) Epilepsy

As discussed briefly in the previous chapter, patients undergoing epilepsy surgery range from infants to those in their late sixties who suffer with "medically intractable" or "medically refractory" epilepsy. For individuals such as these, who constitute approximately 30–35 percent of the population with epilepsy, medications have failed to adequately control their debilitating seizures. Individuals with intractable epilepsy usually suffer from one or more seizure types or have a brain abnormality that can be revealed through neurological examination or imaging studies. However, about a third of patients have a single seizure type and have no definitive abnormality on imaging studies. Additional factors that increase the risk of intractable epilepsy include a long history of active epilepsy and frequent seizures.

Twenty years ago most patients who suffered with medically refractory epilepsy usually struggled with several ineffective medications for years— even decades—before being considered for surgery. Nowadays, most surgeries are performed on patients whose seizures have remained uncontrolled for two to three years, but we know that many good candidates still are being operated on after one or two decades of seizures.

The decision regarding the exact type and number of medications to try, and for how long is determined on a case-by-case basis, as there are no set criteria or an exact formula. For example, if an individual's seizures are frequent, relatively short trials of medication can show the likelihood that anti-epileptic drugs (AEDs) will not help, and surgery may be considered within months. However, if a person's seizures are infrequent, a longer trial is needed to properly determine that the therapy is ineffective.

Alternatively, when epilepsy results from a brain abnormality, such as a tumor or a stroke, fewer AED trials are needed before considering epilepsy surgery since the chances for seizure control with medication in those cases are relatively small. In general, patients are treated with at least two individual anticonvulsant drugs and with a combination of two or more drugs before their epilepsy can be classified as medically refractory and surgery can be considered a viable option. Each of these medication trials must be adequate; that is, the drugs must be increased gradually to the maximally tolerated dose before they are determined ineffective and subsequently discontinued. Candidates for surgery should keep a good record of their AEDs regimens, including the maximal doses, blood levels, and any side effects of each. In practice, however, most neurologists will try at least five or six medications in addition to other treatments such as ketogenic or similar diets, etc., before they consider surgery.

The Risks of Uncontrolled Epilepsy

A person whose seizures persist despite three or more adequate AED trials is unfortunately unlikely to achieve complete seizure control with any new AED. A large and important study published in the *New England Journal of Medicine* several years ago showed that once a person failed three drugs, there was only a 1–2 percent chance of achieving seizure freedom with each new medication. In such cases, the risks and benefits of undergoing surgery should be weighed against the costs of continued seizures and high doses of medication. Many people fail to consider the practical consequences of ongoing seizures and continued high doses of AEDs.

Either alone or in combination, uncontrolled seizures and AEDs can do considerable harm to a person's intellectual, psychological, and social well being, as well as his or her general quality of life. Some evidence suggests that the earlier surgery is performed, the better the outcome will be because early surgery can reduce this burden of medication and seizures over many years or decades. This is especially a consideration in children and young adults whose brains are undergoing important changes in the first decades of life.

Medical Risks of Uncontrolled Epilepsy

The medical risks of persistent, uncontrolled seizures can be placed into one of several broad categories: bodily injury, brain injury, and death. Seizures can cause direct bodily injury, such as lacerations, bruises, fractures, and burns, as well as internal injuries. For example, if a seizure causes a person to fall, he or she might fracture a bone or suffer a laceration of the skin. If the seizure happens while driving, for example, or while engaged in a comparable activity, a more serious and unpredictable injury might occur. Furthermore, tonic-clonic (grand mal) seizures may place physical stress on certain parts of the body, which can cause bone fractures and dislocations as well as induce heart damage among other risks.

One of the most debated issues in the field of epilepsy is whether seizures cause brain damage or not. There is no question that prolonged generalized seizures (status epilepticus) may cause brain, as well as organ, injury. However, the question is whether focal and limited seizures, if uncontrolled, can also cause permanent brain injury. Recent evidence suggests that chemical changes in the brain take place following repeated seizures, eventually leading to nerve cell loss and brain tissue scarring. The exact mechanism by which this occurs is still unknown, but two possibilities are under investigation: Either the excessive release of certain chemicals in the brain or the reduced levels of oxygen in the blood inflicts the resulting brain damage.

Lastly, people who suffer from uncontrolled seizures are at a greater risk of dying than people whose seizures are controlled. The reasons for this are not fully understood, but it is known that about half of these excess deaths are from rather ordinary causes, such as pneumonia, heart disease, and cancer. The other half of these deaths belongs in the category of *sudden unexplained death in epilepsy* (SUDEP). It is believed that SUDEP is caused by either respiratory arrest or heart rhythm abnormalities, both of which may occur either during a seizure or in its aftermath. Among people who have intractable epilepsy, the rate of SUDEP may be as high as 9 per 1,000 patient years. This means that, over the course of a decade, some patients have a 9 percent chance of dying from SUDEP. Compare that with the 0.1 percent risk of death from epilepsy surgery. Furthermore, evidence suggests that the risk of death in patients who have successful surgery (with complete seizure control after surgery) becomes lower, reverting back to that of the general population of patients with epilepsy.

Cognitive and Psychosocial Risks

Uncontrolled seizures and AEDs can also affect cognitive activities, causing poor academic performance, compromised education, and inability to work or drive. For some people with uncontrolled seizures, epilepsy is a progressive disorder with problems affecting memory, mood, and other functions that gradually grow worse over time. AEDs can also adversely affect mental and physical health, leading to significant impairments in quality of life.

The psychosocial risks of uncontrolled epilepsy are also manifold. People are more apt to experience depression, anxiety, and other psychological problems when seizures occur on a frequent basis. This may be due to several factors, including changes in neuronal communication, variations in brain chemistry, and behavioral setbacks (e.g., losing a job because of a seizure). People with uncontrolled seizures can also experience a variety of social problems, including social isolation and stigma. The degree of educational achievement is often lower, and the inability to drive limits independence. These restrictions can result in further constraints on social activities and employment. People with uncontrolled seizures are also less likely to marry, and they earn, on average, less money than people whose seizures are controlled. When children have seizures, parents naturally tend to be overprotective, and this behavior can alter psychological development by restricting independence and natural growth.

Evidence suggests that successful surgery can reverse some of these detrimental effects. After surgery, patients are more likely to alter their marital status, earn more money, drive a vehicle, and engage in a wider range of social activities than people who continue to have uncontrolled seizures. It is also important to note that for young children who are surgery candidates (about 20 percent of children with epilepsy), earlier surgery improves the likelihood of psychosocial and cognitive improvement. Because a child's brain is still forming and developing, it has the greatest potential for recovery.

Who Is a Candidate for Epilepsy Surgery?

The basic principle that both patients and medical professionals should be aware off is that any patient who continues to have seizures despite optimal medical treatment is a potential candidate for surgery. However, as we know, many patients, despite having intractable epilepsy, are not optimal surgical candidates because their seizures are unlikely to benefit from any kind of surgery. What determines who is a surgical candidate or not is not rigid, nor is it determined by a single set of criteria. Furthermore, the criteria by which centers determine who is or not a surgical candidate vary considerably between hospitals, national health systems, neurologist, neurosurgeons, and countries, and it is very much influenced by medical and general culture, medical systems, economics, religion, and more.

In general, the criteria listed here serve as a starting point of reference. Any patient with the following characteristics is a potential candidate:

- Disabling seizures
- Medically intractable epilepsy
- Focal seizures arising from one brain area
- Seizures that cause alterations in consciousness or memory

It is important to stress that a patient doesn't need to have all of the above characteristics to be considered for surgery. Again, every patient is unique in this respect. Let's discuss some of these criteria in more details. Seizures that lead people to consider surgery are usually those that cause alterations or loss of awareness or consciousness (also known as "complex partial" seizures). These seizures have the most potential to cause serious injury and impair quality of life. Most commonly, people who have surgery have either complex partial or secondarily generalized tonic-clonic (grand mal). Partial seizures are the most common type of epilepsy treated with surgery because they begin in a defined brain region. Secondarily generalized seizures are also operable because the focus can be isolated and removed, usually resulting in the complete elimination or drastic reduction of seizures. Complex partial seizures, by virtue of interrupting or altering consciousness, have the most adverse psychosocial and medical repercussions. Additionally, some seizures, although they might not cause loss of awareness (simple partial seizures), might be so unpleasant or upsetting that surgery could still be considered as an option. For example, a seizure that periodically gives rise to intense nausea and vomiting or one that leads to socially unacceptable behavior might warrant consideration of surgery.

In spite of this, it is clear that many patients with focal seizures without changes in awareness are also candidates for surgery. I have seen many patients over the years who had, for example, focal motor seizures (seizures causing only motor manifestations such as jerking of a leg, arm, or hand) or purely sensory seizures (in which there is pain or numbness on one limb or body area) who were operated because the seizures were socially or psychologically disabling.

Although the number of seizures per week or month tends to have considerable weight on the decision to proceed or not with surgery, the number of seizures per se should not be viewed as critical. At one end of the spectrum are those patients with daily or weekly seizures and, for those, surgery should always be the first choice. In the middle of the spectrum are the vast majority of patients we operate. Although most people who elect to undergo surgery have seizures at least once per month or every other month, others have many fewer seizures and surgery is indicated. For example, a person who has just one or two seizures per year may not, as a result, be able to drive. Other patients have very few seizures per year, but they may be severe and serious each and every time they occur. However infrequently, they pose a real danger to life. For example, several years ago I treated a patient who had one single cluster of seizures per year; however, every time she had seizures, she ended up in the intensive care unit with a tube in her lungs, medical complications, and a long recovery time. Individuals like this, who have very few seizures per year, are still candidates as long as they meet other criteria for surgery.

Last, it is important to consider the predictability of seizures. If an individual suffers from only nocturnal (while asleep) seizures, he or she may still drive an automobile and live a relatively unrestricted life. However, an individual who suffers from erratically occurring seizures may be more inclined to consider surgery. In general, the affected individual and/or family are the only ones who can state with certainty whether the symptoms of uncontrolled seizures are intolerable enough to consider surgical treatment.

Epilepsy surgery can also be especially beneficial to patients who have seizures associated with structural brain abnormalities, such as benign brain tumors, malformations of blood vessels (including arteriovenous malformations, cavernous, or venous angiomas), and strokes. Surgery in these cases may be utilized for two reasons: to control the seizures and/or to remove the abnormality in the brain. In many cases, the area adjacent to the abnormal tissue may in fact be the origin of the seizures. The part of the brain where the seizure begins often provides no useful functions. Removing this abnormal tissue may lead to improvement or complete control of the seizures.

Finally, patients with severe and frequent seizures associated with falls may benefit from sectioning of the corpus callosum. This surgery is intended to be palliative (helps but doesn't cure) and is discussed later on.

Who Is Not a Candidate for Epilepsy Surgery?

Epilepsy surgery is an elective procedure for the vast majority of patients. Therefore, patients whose epilepsy is relatively benign and easy to control are, in principle, not candidates. For these individuals, surgery has potentially more risks than potential benefits. However, as stated earlier, the severity of epilepsy is largely a subjective matter, and for physicians to make decisions based on their views and beliefs can potentially deprive some patients from curative procedures. Thus, it is always best for the patient and the family to ask and discuss with more than one physician if surgery should be considered.

The following list represents situations in which epilepsy surgery is usually not a viable option:

- Patients who have poor compliance to medical treatment are not good candidates for surgery because of their unreliability in following medical advice.
- Patients with severe medical conditions that significantly increase the risk of surgery.
- Patients with primary generalized epilepsy are not candidates for epilepsy surgery because there is no specific localized focus that can be isolated and removed in such cases. These patients generally tend to do well with AEDs, and medical treatment can control more than 80 percent of seizures.
- As stated earlier, anyone with focal epilepsy is a potential candidate for surgery in principle. However, the location of the seizure area may, at times, make resective surgery impossible or likely to cause unacceptable deficits. Additionally, an important aspect of epilepsy surgery involves "functional mapping"—testing different areas of the brain before an area is removed to be sure that it is safe for removal. If an individual's seizures originate from an area that is too close to the regions of the brain that control speech or memory, he or she may not be a candidate for surgery, no matter how precisely the focus is located. Or, for example, if the focus is located in the vision center, the outcome may be unacceptable vision loss, which results in losing half the vision. Sometimes a surgeon may be able to remove a portion of the abnormal tissue in order to reduce the frequency of the seizures even if he or she cannot remove the entire area.
- People who have multiple focal (multifocal) areas causing epilepsy may make focal surgery likely to fail and are not good candidates for surgery.
- The type of epilepsy disorder a person has may influence the

decision to consider surgery. Some types of epilepsy are known to disappear over time. In such a case, it would be inappropriate to perform surgery for a condition that will remit in the near future, such as benign rolandic epilepsy. Other types of epilepsy are believed to have a progressive downhill course, such as progressive myoclonic epilepsy or aggressive malignant brain tumor, so surgery would certainly not afford any long-term benefit and should not be performed.

- People who have non-epileptic seizures, episodes that resemble epileptic seizures but are not. Individuals with non-epileptic seizures do not respond to treatment with AEDs and are certainly not candidates for surgery because their attacks do not stem from epileptic activity in the brain. Instead, patients with non-epileptic seizures must enter into therapy with a psychiatrist or psychologist in the hopes of identifying and treating the underlying psychosocial stress that causes their episodes to occur.
- Patients with severe psychiatric disorders such as long-standing psychosis are also not candidates for epilepsy surgery. Here, it is important to state that many patients with intractable epilepsy and more recent psychosis could be considered for surgery as the psychosis may be directly caused by the seizures. It is in patients with chronic or long-term psychosis where surgery will be not recommended.

Some patients who are not candidates for traditional resective surgery for any of the listed reasons may be candidates for other treatments, such as the vagus nerve stimulator (VNS) or responsive neurostimulator (RNS) (see Chapter 5).

In the end, the decision to have surgery is subject to and influenced by many medical, psychological, social, and cultural factors. It is a balance between the risk and benefits of surgery versus persistent long-term and maybe lifetime epilepsy. Careful preoperative counseling should always accompany a patient's decision so that he or she can be fully informed of the risks and benefits associated with surgery.

CHAPTER THREE
THE EVALUATION: WHICH TESTS ARE NEEDED BEFORE SURGERY?

- The pre-surgical evaluation aims to establish a likelihood of seizure control after surgery while minimizing the disruption of normal brain functioning.
- Proper patient selection and thorough pre-surgical testing are the building blocks of surgical success.
- The types of tests that make up each patient's pre-surgical evaluation depend on the patient's specific type of epilepsy and the surgery being considered.
- The tests most often performed as part of the pre-surgical evaluation are the electroencephalogram (EEG), video EEG, brain magnetic resonance imaging (MRI), and neuropsychological examination.
- Less frequent tests include positron emission tomography with fludeoxyglucose (PET-FDG), magnetoencephalogram (MEG), single photon emission computed tomography (SPECT), functional MRI (fMRI), and the Wada test.

Once both the patient and physician decide together to consider surgical treatment, the patient must undergo inpatient and outpatient medical testing. This testing may be quite time-consuming and spread out over several months. The purpose of these tests is to accurately identify the abnormal area or areas of the brain causing the seizures. Additionally, the tests are necessary to determine whether surgery will impact any areas of the brain that control important functions such as language, memory, and movement. Thus, the pre-surgical evaluation aims to maximize seizure control after surgery while also eliminating or minimizing the disruption of normal brain functioning. Success rates for epilepsy surgery are constantly improving due to advances in preoperative assessments. Proper patient selection combined with careful pre-surgical testing are the building blocks of surgical success.

There Is No "Silver Bullet" Test in Epilepsy Surgery

No single test can show physicians everything they need to know before suggesting epilepsy surgery. Thus, compiling information from a wide range of sources is needed to accurately and safely determine what type of surgery to perform and which area(s) of the brain to target. The types of tests that comprise each patient's pre-surgical evaluation depend on the specific type of epilepsy observed and the subsequent surgery being considered. However, the procedures utilized to determine pre-surgical candidacy can be grouped into three main categories:

1. Those that are always performed (Absolutely needed).
2. Those that are frequently performed (Often needed).
3. Those that are sometimes performed (Sometimes needed).

History and Physical Exam

Despite all the amazing advances in medical technology, nothing surpasses the importance of the history and physical examination by the neurologist or epilepsy specialist. This part of the evaluation establishes the seizure type(s), assesses the potential causes of the seizure disorder, and helps the physician arrive at the precise diagnosis and prognosis. After administering a history and physical examination, an experienced physician can usually determine whether surgery is a good option. The history and physical often contain important clues regarding the area of the brain that might be causing the seizures; sometimes, a physician can even form a preliminary opinion as to the potential risks or benefits of surgery.

A doctor may begin the evaluation by asking about a patient's birth and development. For example, any difficulties that occurred during the mother's pregnancy and/or the patient's delivery may indicate an early injury to the brain or an abnormality of brain development that could have resulted in the seizure disorder.

The physician will then perform a physical examination to ensure that a patient's seizures are not resulting from a medical disorder, such as an underlying chemical or rare genetic disorder. The physician will also ask if there was any lack of sleep, unusual stress, or recent illnesses that could have provoked the patient's seizures. Additionally, a neurological examination will be performed to evaluate mental, muscle, and sensory function. If neurological symptoms such as memory difficulty, weakness of one arm or leg, walking difficulty, or visual disturbances are present, it may reveal abnormal activity in a particular region of the brain.

A detailed assessment of a patient's seizure history may provide many important clues as well. The physician will ask questions with regards to the seizure type, seizure frequency, and the patient's responses to specific medications, all to better and more accurately pinpoint where the seizures might start. If the patient or a witness can describe in detail what exactly happens before, during, and after a seizure, this information can be invaluable to the physician. The specific symptoms a patient may exhibit immediately prior to a seizure (aura) or while a seizure is occurring may indicate where the abnormal epileptic discharge begins in the brain. For example, a seizure beginning with tingling in one hand usually starts in the opposite parietal lobe. Visual symptoms, such as flashing lights or colors, suggest that seizures originate in the occipital lobe or visual area. In contrast, a seizure that begins with a feeling of déjà vu or fear often originates in the temporal or frontal lobe. Seizures that cause lip smacking often arise in a temporal lobe, while the stiffening of one side of the body might indicate that the seizure began on the opposite side of the brain. Considered together, the symptoms, history, and physical exam may provide clues about the likely source or region involved in the generation of the seizures.

Electroencephalogram (EEG)
The brain produces electrical activity that may be analyzed using an EEG machine. The EEG is a safe and painless procedure, in which 16–21 electrodes are attached to a patient's scalp with removable glue. Before beginning the process, EEG technicians sometimes measure the head first in order to place the electrodes accurately. The electrodes are then connected by wires to an electrical box, which is in turn connected to the EEG machine. Once everything is in place, the EEG displays the brain's electrical activity on a computer screen or on graph paper (Fig. 3, pg. 28). The electrodes measure the patient's brain waves and detect any abnormal electrical discharges, as well as the location of those discharges. The information collected by the EEG can help physicians to pinpoint exactly where epileptic brain activity begins.

Because the EEG usually records *interictal activity*, or the brain activity between seizures (ictal activity means activity during a seizure), a person with epilepsy might have a normal EEG at any time. Seizures occupy a tiny percentage of a patient's life, and the EEG can be taken during the large majority of time in which seizures do not occur.

Additionally, abnormal areas may go undetected by the EEG if the activity arises from deep regions "outside the reach" of the scalp electrodes or if the volume of brain affected is too small to generate abnormal waves of sufficient size.

To increase the probability that the EEG captures epileptic activity, there are several techniques physicians utilize to induce a seizure. These techniques include sleep deprivation (the patient may be asked to sleep only a few hours before the EEG), hyperventilation (the patient is asked to breathe heavily and quickly, usually for about 3 minutes), photosensitivity (the patient may be shown strobe lights), and the administering of certain medications or alcohol (during a hospital stay, adult patients may be asked to take specific medications or drink alcohol).

An outpatient routine EEG done at a hospital or clinic may be as short as 30 minutes to an hour. During a "take-home" or "ambulatory" EEG, which usually lasts between 24 to 72 hours, the electrodes attached to the patient's head are connected to a portable computer that the patient brings home. The computer records any seizure activity from the electrodes. Throughout the procedure, the patient is asked to keep an activity log that lists the times at which he or she eats, drinks, or engages in other activities.

To prepare for any EEG, the patient can help by washing his or her hair the night before the day of the test. However, the patient should avoid using conditioners, hair creams, sprays, or styling gels.

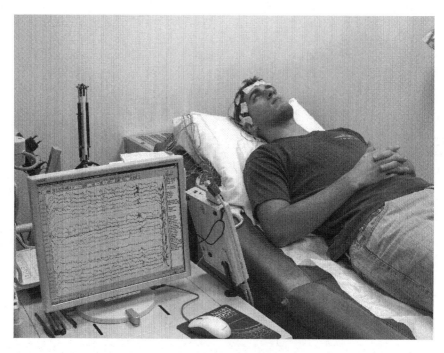

Figure 3: Patient undergoing an EEG test.
(Dr. Ruben Kuzniecky/NYU)

Video-EEG

To gather more evidence for seizure localization before surgery, most physicians prefer to record and observe seizures using video EEG. In fact, most consider VEEG studies necessary for all patients before surgery because surprises can occur. VEEG studies are done in the setting of a specialized epilepsy-monitoring unit in a hospital, during which electrodes are usually glued to the scalp using very strong and smelly glue called *collodion*. EEG and video are recorded continuously for many days so that patient's behavior (auditory and visual) during seizures can be observed along with the electrical activity occurring in the brain at the same time (Fig. 4, pg. 30). Trained nurses or EEG technologists can also perform testing during the seizure.

Because seizures may occur relatively infrequently in some people, AEDs are often reduced in order to provoke seizures. This dose reduction may lead to seizures being stronger than usual, so close observation is required. Intravenous (IV) access is sometimes established when medications are stopped in order to ensure the rapid delivery of medication if a seizure must be stopped quickly. Another seizure trigger is sleep deprivation or changes in sleep patterns. This is often done to provoke events. Patients may be admitted to the hospital for a few days or up to several weeks, depending on how often their seizures occur and how many need to be studied. Physicians usually need to analyze several seizures to fully ascertain which side and lobe of the brain are responsible for the seizures.

A patient who is going to have VEEG monitoring should bring clothing to the hospital that can be buttoned, instead of pullovers. The patient should also bring reading materials, video games, and/or computers to keep busy because a hospital stay can be quite boring. After the EEG, a silicone substance is applied to the electrodes to remove the collodion. In the event that the adhesive is not completely removed, hot oil hair treatment (like VO5) can be used to remove the remainder.

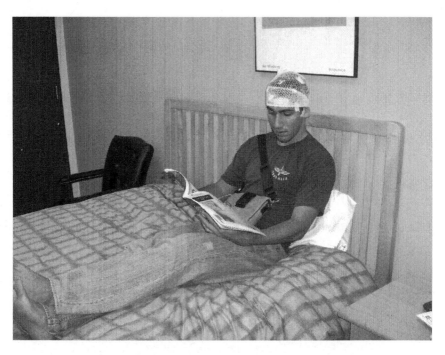
Figure 4: Video EEG study done for seizure characterization. The patient is admitted to the hospital and undergoes EEG with video.
(Dr. Ruben Kuzniecky, NYU)

Magnetic Resonance Imaging

MRI provides detailed images of the brain's structure. The MRI uses a powerful magnet that changes the spin on atomic particles and then measures the changes in the magnetic field as the particles resume their previous course. These changes create an image of the brain that can be analyzed for any structural abnormalities that may be associated with seizures, such as strokes, tumors, blood vessel abnormalities, birth defects, and scar tissue from traumatic injury. In temporal lobe epilepsy, which is the most common type of epilepsy treated with surgery, shrinkage of a part of the lobe located deep within the brain (the hippocampus) can be seen.

The MRI exam involves a patient lying very still within a large, powerful, circular magnet. The machine makes loud noises in different sequences throughout the exam, but these should not be too troublesome for the patient. The MRI is safe and painless, but most machines confine the patient's head and upper body to a small place (Fig. 5, pg. 32).

Individuals with claustrophobia (fear of small places), and many who never knew they were claustrophobic can become frightened when they see or experience the confined space. Medications for relaxation can be given if needed (children often require sedation). Occasionally, a contrast material will be injected into the patient as part of the MRI examination to improve clarity in the scanned images. A typical MRI takes between 30 and 45 minutes, including the time for patient positioning, preparations, and scanning.

Because of the MRI's strong magnet, individuals with cardiac pacemakers, metal heart valves, or any other bodies should generally not undergo an MRI scan.

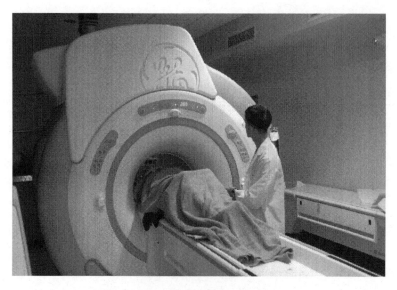

Figure 5:Patient undergoing MRI scan.
(Unknown Author [Public Domain]/National Institute of Mental Health)

Neuropsychological Testing

Neuropsychologists are interested in how seizures affect the way a person with epilepsy thinks and remembers. Neuropsychological testing consists of a complex battery of tests that look at IQ, memory (both verbal and nonverbal), learning capability, and mental flexibility, as well as an assessment of emotional and personality traits. This testing can last from 4 to 6 hours. The neuropsychologist analyzes this information in order to characterize cognitive and emotional function. The patient's results are compared with the results of people in the same age range and of similar background. In the written report, recommendations for further treatment, job retraining, or retesting may be included. In some cases, the neuropsychologist may be able to determine if a region of the patient's brain is not functioning normally. Sometimes this region is also the place where seizures are originating.

As part of the examination, the neuropsychologist will also determine the patient's emotional well-being and social support system. Any potential problems are addressed before surgery is performed.

Procedures That Are Frequently Performed

The following procedures are frequently, but not always, performed on patients as part of their pre-surgical evaluation. Physicians decide on a case-by-case basis whether any or all of these procedures are necessary to supplement the previous examinations. These procedures include: computed tomography (CT), functional magnetic resonance imaging (fMRI), magnetic resonance spectroscopy (MRS), positron emission tomography (PET), single-photon emission computed tomography (SPECT), and magnetoencephalography (MEG).

Computed Tomography

CT (or CAT scan) was introduced in the early 1970s. It revolutionized the practice of neurology and neurosurgery by letting doctors see inside the brain without surgery for the first time. The CT scan is normal for most people with epilepsy. It is also utilized to see structural abnormalities including atrophy (shrinking of the brain), scar tissue, strokes, tumors, or abnormal blood vessels. Just like ordinary x-rays, CT scans expose the patient to radiation. However, the amount is low and the procedure is considered safe, even if it needs to be repeated several times. The scanner is a large machine, and it is less confining for patients than an MRI machine

(Fig. 6, pg. 35). The advantages of CT scanning include speed and easy availability in most places. However, it has lower resolution than MRI for showing brain structures, especially abnormalities and, for this reason, it is rarely used today as part of the pre-surgical evaluation.

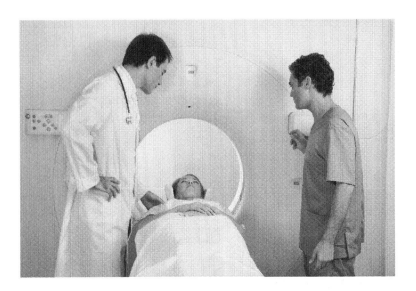

Figure 6: Patient undergoing CT scan.
(Tyler Olson/Shutterstock)

Functional MRI

Functional MRI can be useful for some people who are going on to have epilepsy surgery. The fMRI uses magnetic resonance imaging to measure the quick, tiny changes that take place in an active part of the brain. It can identify regions where blood vessels are expanding, chemical changes are taking place, or extra oxygen is being delivered—all signs that this part of the brain is currently processing information and giving commands to the body. Physicians know the general areas of the brain that control speech, sensation, memory, and other functions. However, the exact locations vary from individual to individual, and even injuries and disease, such as a stroke or a brain tumor, can cause functions to shift to other parts of the brain. An fMRI can help determine which part of the brain is handling critical functions. By localizing these functions, a surgeon can make sure to avoid removing during surgery those parts of the brain that are vital to a patient (Fig. 7, pg. 37).

In an fMRI, the patient performs particular tasks, such as reading, speaking, and moving his or her fingers, while the imaging is taking place. The fMRI records the changes taking place in the area of the brain responsible for these tasks. By performing specific tasks that correspond to different functions, the fMRI can locate the part of the brain that controls that function. This information can then be incorporated into a surgical planner to help a surgeon avoid these areas. Despite the fact that fMRI has been available for a few years, the information it provides still has to be compared with other standard tests carefully.

Depending on how many images are needed, the exam generally takes anywhere from 15 to 45 minutes, although a very detailed study may take longer. Patients are asked not to move during the actual imaging process, but some movement is allowed between sequences. Since fMRI uses the same machine as an MRI, the standard preparations for an MRI procedure are necessary. Individuals with cardiac pacemakers, metal heart valves, or other metal in their bodies should generally not have an fMRI scan.

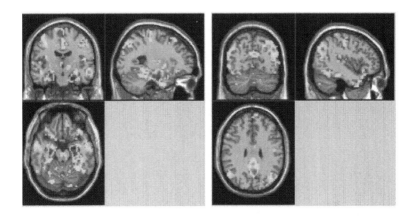

Figure 7: Examples of fMRI scans.
(Dr. Ruben Kuzniecky, NYU)

Magnetic Resonance Spectroscopy

The nuclei of certain atoms have physical qualities called resonance frequencies, which provide chemical information. MRS examines those atoms to determine the amounts of specific chemical compounds in the brain, such as neurotransmitters and energy supplies. This information can provide clues to the causes and effects of epilepsy. MRS may also help to identify areas of the brain from which seizures originate, but currently this particular use is only considered investigational.

An MRS exam usually takes about 60 minutes, and it uses the same machine as the fMRI and the MRI. Therefore, the same precautions that are necessary for the MRI and fMRI should be observed for the MRS procedure.

Positron Emission Tomography

PET, also called a "PET scan," generates images based on the detection of positrons—tiny particles emitted from a very low and safe dose of radioactive substance administered to the patient—so as to show the chemical functioning of brain tissue. The PET images obtained while a patient is not having seizures can also provide information to pinpoint the region of the brain that is the source of the epilepsy.

Before the examination begins, a radioactive substance produced in a machine called a *cyclotron* is attached or tagged to a natural body compound. Usually this compound is glucose (a form of sugar), but sometimes it can be water or ammonia. A PET scanner has a hole in the middle and resembles a large doughnut. Inside the machine are multiple rings of detectors that record the energy emissions from the radioactive substance in the patient's body and subsequently produce an image.

The different colors or degrees of brightness seen in a PET image represent the different levels of tissue or organ function. For example, healthy tissue that uses a large amount of glucose for energy accumulates some of the tagged compound, which is reflected as a bright region in the PET images (Fig. 8, pg. 40). On the other hand, unhealthy tissue, such as the tissue that triggers seizures, uses less glucose for energy and appears less bright in the PET images.

A PET scan is usually performed on an outpatient basis. Patients are asked not to eat for 4 hours before the scan, but they are encouraged to drink water. If a patient is taking regular medication, he or she may be asked to discontinue that medication just before the test. Diabetic patients, specifically, should ask for strict diet guidelines so as to control glucose levels during the day of the test.

During the PET exam, the patient will lie down on an examination table and be given the radioactive substance as an IV injection (in some cases, it will be given through an existing IV line or inhaled as a gas). It takes approximately 30 to 60 minutes for the substance to travel through the patient's body and be absorbed by the tissue under study. During this time, the patient will rest in a partially darkened room and avoid significant moving or talking because this could alter the localization of the administered substance. After this resting time, the scanning will begin and will usually take an additional 30 to 45 minutes.

The disadvantages of PET include the cost of the procedure, the short-lived radioactive exposure, and the limited number of scanners available. However, PET is very sensitive in patients with temporal lobe epilepsy and can significantly aid in the decision-making process on route to surgery. As a result of the use of radioactive compounds, patients who are pregnant or nursing cannot undergo this procedure.

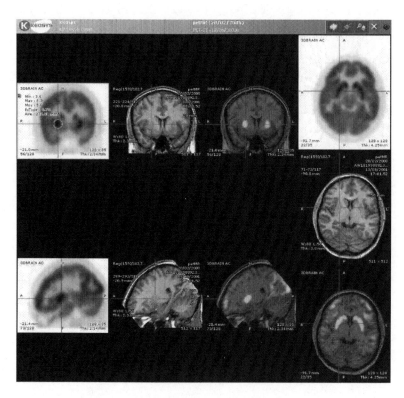

Figure 8: Examples of PET scans and MRI scans.
(Mco44 at en.wikipedia [Public domain]/Wikimedia Commons)

Single-Photon Emission Computed Tomography

Like PET, a SPECT scan involves injecting a low, safe dose of a radioactive tracer into patients. The particles that this tracer emits are used to create an image of the brain. The images produced by a SPECT exam show how blood flows within the brain, with different colors representing different levels of blood flow (Fig. 9, pg. 42). Simply put, the more blood that flows through a certain region, the more particles are emitted. SPECT scans, like PET scans, may be done between seizures, but they can also be used during seizures. A SPECT obtained during or immediately after a seizure (seconds to minutes) may be particularly useful for pinpointing a seizure focus because it may show increased blood flow in the area where seizures arise. However, the injection of radioactive tracer must take place very early during or after the seizure in order to reliably localize the responsible brain region, which can be very difficult to accomplish.

New computer techniques allow physicians to measure the differences between SPECT scans taken during and between seizures in order to obtain "subtraction" SPECT images. These images can be superimposed onto the patient's MRI to pinpoint the seizure origin. This technique may be most helpful when seizures begin outside the temporal lobe and MRI scans do not show a structural abnormality. Additionally, SPECT scans are cheaper and more readily available than the higher resolution PET scans but are less sensitive than PET.

During a SPECT scan, the patient will receive an injection of a small amount of a radioactive compound. The compound is a chemical tracer that travels through the blood stream, taking about 10 to 20 seconds to reach the brain. Then a special camera will rotates around the patient's head and take images for about 30 to 45 minutes. A computer collects the information emitted by the radioactive compound and translates them into 2-dimensional images. These images are then added together to form a 3-dimensional picture of the brain.

As with PET, patients who are pregnant or nursing should not undergo a SPECT scan. After a SPECT scan, patients should drink plenty of fluids to flush out any tracer left in their bodies.

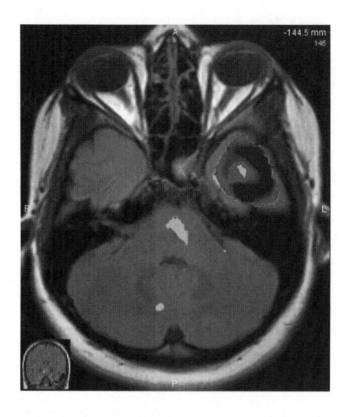

Figure 9: SPECT scan showing blood flow increase corresponding to seizure onset.
(Dr. Ruben Kuzniecky, NYU)

Magnetoencephalogrophy

The same electrical currents that generate EEG output also produce small magnetic fields. These magnetic fields are measured in a special device called the magnetoencephalograph, or MEG, which is placed with the patient in a specially designed room that is shielded from external electrical sources. To some degree, MEG is similar to EEG. However, an important difference is that the skull and the tissue surrounding the brain affect the magnetic fields measured by MEG much less than they affect the electrical impulses measured by EEG. Therefore, MEG has greater accuracy than EEG owing to the minimal distortion of the signal (Fig. 10, pg. 45).

MEG is usually performed simultaneously with EEG. It can be used to localize the area from which seizures originate as well as pinpoint the sites of vital brain functions such as touch, vision, movement, and language. In some cases, an MRI scan may show a lesion, but the EEG findings are not entirely consistent with the MRI information. An MEG may be able to confirm that the epileptic activity is indeed arising from the lesion, and a decision can then be made regarding surgery. Additionally, for patients who have brain tumors or other lesions, MEG may be able to map the exact location of the normally functioning areas near the lesion. Surgery can then be properly planned to minimize postoperative weakness or loss of brain function.

Last, in patients who have had past brain surgery, the electrical field measured by EEG may be distorted by the changes in scalp and brain anatomy. If further surgery is being considered, MEG may be able to provide necessary information without more invasive EEG studies.

No special preparations are required for MEG, unless sedation is planned. In that case, the patient may be asked to refrain from eating anything after midnight on the day of the exam, and regular medicines should be taken with a little bit of water. A patient going in for MEG should wear loose, comfortable clothing. He or she should not wear jewelry, hair spray, make-up, hearing aids, or removable dental work. Any patients with a vagus nerve stimulator (see Chapter 5) may be able to have an MEG study using special filters.

During an MEG, a few EEG electrodes are glued around the patient's head, while one is placed over the patient's heart. Three small coils are taped to the forehead, and two more are attached to earplugs. The patient will lie down on the MEG bed, where a small metal coil will touch all of the different dots around the patient's head to record its shape. As soon as this information is entered into the computer, the MEG study can begin. Sensors are then placed over the patient's head, but they do not cover the patient's face. The coils and EEG electrodes are plugged into these sensors. The MEG exam takes from anywhere between 1 and 2.5 hours. During this time, the patient is asked to lie as still as possible. Sometimes stimulation tests are performed as part of the MEG exam. In these cases, little plastic sensors are placed onto the patient's fingers, or the patient is shown a video with different colors. This allows the physician to determine which part of the patient's brain controls movement and sensory functions. In general, MEG is less used than the other techniques because it is expensive, and very specialized machines and personnel are needed. Also, there are very few MEG machines when compared with MRI or PET.

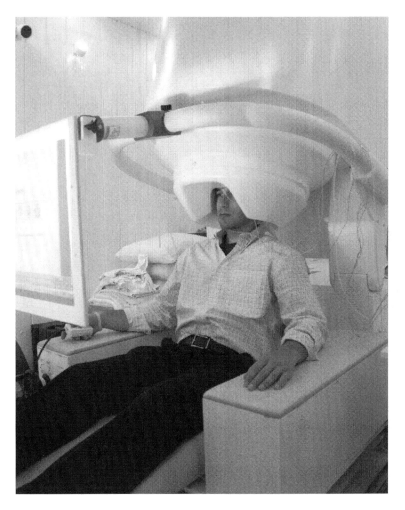

Figure 10: Patient undergoing MEG exam.
(Unknown National Institute of Mental Health Author
[Public Domain]/Wikimedia Commons)

Procedures That Are Sometimes Performed

The following procedures are rarely performed on patients as part of their preliminary pre-surgical evaluation. Instead, they are usually reserved for those patients who have already been evaluated through a variety of previous examinations and are being seriously considered for surgery by the entire epilepsy team. Patients who are evaluated using these procedures will almost always continue on to have surgery. These procedures include the intracarotid sodium amobarbital (Wada) test, intracranial electroencephalography (IEEG), and cortical mapping.

Intracarotid Sodium Amobarbital (Wada) Test

The intracarotid sodium amobarbital test is called a "Wada test," named after Dr. Juh Wada, a Japanese neurosurgeon who first performed it. The Wada test assesses memory and language functions by inducing one hemisphere of the brain to sleep with a short-acting anesthetic, such as amobarbital, and studying to what degree functions are still working in the other awake hemisphere. The Wada test is not necessarily required as part of the pre-surgical evaluation, and different epilepsy centers have different criteria for determining when it is used. The test takes about 2 hours and is done on an outpatient basis.

The procedure begins with a cerebral angiogram to determine the brain's blood flow patterns and to make sure that there are no obstacles to performing the Wada. A neuroradiologist inserts a catheter (a long, narrow tube) into an artery, usually in the upper thigh. A local anesthetic numbs the area, and a needle is inserted into the artery. The tube is threaded through the needle, and the needle is then removed. The catheter is guided up to either the right or left internal carotid artery in the neck, the artery that supplies the brain with blood. Once the catheter is in place, a contrast dye is injected. Some patients report a warm sensation when this happens, or a momentary vision of flashing lights. The injected dye can be seen on a special x-ray machine, which takes pictures of the dye as it flows through the blood vessels of the brain. Once the angiogram is completed, the catheter stays in place for the Wada.

Before an angiogram, a patient should not eat for about 8 hours. He or she may also take steroid (cortisone) tablets to reduce brain swelling. These tablets can sometimes cause upset stomach issues, so a patient who has previously had a stomach ulcer should notify his or her physician accordingly.

During the Wada test, the neuroradiologist will alternate putting each side of the brain to sleep for a few minutes each. This is done by injecting sodium amobarbital (also called sodium amytal) through the catheter into the right or left internal carotid artery. If the right carotid artery is injected, the right side of the brain goes to sleep and cannot communicate with the left side. Subsequently, language and memory can be assessed from the still functioning, non-anesthetized side of the brain. Language (speech) is controlled by only one side of the brain. Therefore, if the left carotid artery is injected and the patient cannot speak, language function must be located on the left side of the patient's brain.

It is known that both sides of the brain can control memory, but the Wada may determine which side of a patient's brain has better memory functioning. For example, while under anesthesia, the patient may be presented with objects, pictures, or words. The side of the brain that is awake tries to recognize and remember what it sees. After the sedative wears off (usually 10 minutes or so after injection) and both sides of the brain are awake once more, the neuropsychologist asks the patient what was shown. If the patient doesn't remember, the items are individually shown to the patient one at a time, and the patient is asked whether he or she saw each one before. The patient's responses are recorded word-for-word. After a resting period, the other side of the brain is put to sleep. To achieve this, the catheter is partly withdrawn and threaded into the internal carotid artery on the other side.

A new angiogram is then performed for that side of the brain. Different objects and pictures are shown to the patient, and the side of the brain that is awake (which was asleep before) tries to recognize and remember what it sees. After the sedative wears off, the patient is asked again what was shown. If the patient doesn't remember, the patient is shown items one at a time and asked if he or she has seen them before. The information collected through this procedure helps to assess the risks of surgery and may also confirm that a temporal lobe is functioning abnormally. If the seizure focus is located in the hemisphere that does not control language and has weaker memory function, this may permit a larger resection of tissue during surgery. If, however, the seizure focus is found to be located in the hemisphere that controls language or the hemisphere that has better memory, the surgeon may require more tests to ensure the patient can safely undergo surgery. Additionally, the surgeon may individually tailor the surgery so as to specifically avoid the brain tissue that controls these vital functions.

A Wada test is generally a safe procedure with very few risks. However, there is a small risk of some complications. These complications can be as minor as pain where the catheter is inserted or as serious as a potential stroke. The risk of a stroke during the cerebral angiogram test is less than 1 percent overall. It is greater, but still relatively low, in older people with atherosclerosis.

Intracranial Electroencephalography

After all the aforementioned studies are performed, the exact origin of seizures may still be uncertain in some patients. The decision to use IEEG depends on the findings from the previous tests. If all evidence points to the same area of the brain as the focus of the seizures, most epilepsy centers proceed to surgery without invasive electrodes. However, if the information is inconsistent or indefinite, or the focus lies in or near functional brain areas, invasive electrodes are often used to provide a more exact localization. These electrodes are inserted by a neurosurgeon with the patient under general anesthesia in the operating room. IEEG, also known as "invasive monitoring," is most commonly done as the first-stage procedure before epilepsy surgery takes place.

The skull prevents most brain waves from reaching the scalp, so sometimes they cannot be picked up and interpreted through regular EEG. Placing the electrodes inside the skull allows the surgeon to get more accurate information regarding the specific area from which the seizures arise and can help the surgeon decide which area(s) of the brain to remove. While the usual clinical EEG electrodes measure the combined activity of millions of brain cells, an IEEG can measure the activity of small groups of brain cells. With these electrodes, it is possible to see the activity in epileptic and normal brain circuits.

There are two main types of electrodes: *subdural* and *depth*. Subdural electrodes are metal electrodes embedded in plastic and arranged as either a strip or a large grid. Grids are rectangular plates varying in size, and are usually no bigger than 8 × 8 cm. Strips are narrower—perhaps 1 cm wide—and range from 4 to 8 cm long (Fig. 11, pg. 50). Both strips and grids cover a large area and record directly from the brain without interference from the scalp and skull. The electrodes are placed on the brain underneath the dura mater (one of the layers of tissue covering the brain). In some cases, the electrodes are inserted through a *burr hole*, a small hole drilled in the skull. In other cases, a portion of the skull is removed, the electrodes are put into place, and the piece of skull is replaced or frozen in a sterile location. After the testing is completed, the piece of skull is replaced. There is a moderate amount of discomfort for several days after subdural electrodes are placed on the brain, and thus medicine is given for pain relief. Depth electrodes are thin, wire-like plastic tubes with metal contact points spread out along their length (Fig. 12, pg. 51). They are inserted through small burr holes into sites situated deep within the brain. These electrodes may be placed on one or both sides of the brain, depending upon need.

The wires of the electrodes are connected to an EEG machine after the head is carefully wrapped with a sterile dressing. Video EEG monitoring can then be performed in the same way as when electrodes are attached to the scalp. Seizures are recorded, and the precise location of their origin can be determined. Although intracranial video EEG recording is needed only for a minority of patients, it is nonetheless essential for some to determine where to operate. It is sometimes safer to use intracranial electrodes than to proceed directly to surgery since better definition of the area to be removed might reduce the chances of producing permanent neurological complication and improve chances of success.

IEEG monitoring, the first stage of surgery, can take as little as several days or as long as several weeks. The second stage of surgery is when the surgeon performs a second operation and first removes the electrodes and then does the resection of the abnormal brain tissue using the information gathered from the electrical recordings. Depending on individual circumstances, surgery might be performed immediately upon concluding the monitoring or up to several weeks later.

Since IEEG is a neurosurgical procedure, it carries the same risks as any brain surgery, including bleeding (less than 1 percent chance), infection (1 percent chance), stroke, and death (1/1000). The major risks of subdural electrodes are infection (which increases during prolonged use, especially after 6 to 8 days), bleeding, and brain swelling. Depth electrodes carry some additional risks, especially bleeding within the brain. However, they are less likely than subdural electrodes to cause infection or brain swelling. Chances of any permanent serious complication with intracranial EEG are small, but the procedure should still only be done when absolutely necessary.

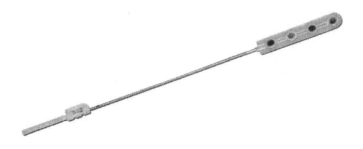

Figure 11: Cortical strip lead used for IEEG.
(Dr. Ruben Kuzniecky/NYU)

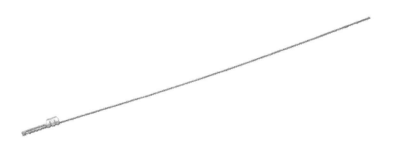

Figure 12: Depth lead used for IEEG.
(Dr. Ruben Kuzniecky/NYU)

Cortical Mapping

When electrodes are placed on the brain for IEEG, they may also be stimulated with a small electrical current to map brain function. The exact location of various functions differs from person to person, and cortical (brain) mapping can help confirm the areas of the brain that control speech, language, memory, sight, and other skills. The mapping procedures involve stimulation of the brain with mild currents to temporarily activate or shut down certain areas. Not all patients, however, require brain mapping. For example, it is not normally done in children under the age of four because they are able to regain most faculties they might lose as a result of surgery. Additionally, since the left side of the brain is primarily responsible for the control of language, patients that need tissue removed from the right side of the brain usually don't require cortical mapping.

At each location within a brain region, the physician starts by applying the lowest possible current with a small electrical probe. Gradually, the current is increased until a preset maximum is reached or until a response is observed. Each location is tested in this way to create an accurate "map" of functions present within that region of the patient's brain.

Areas involved with movement can be identified electrically even if the patient is under anesthesia. For example, if a patient's limbs or face start and stop moving, the area being tested is responsible for movement. However, to map areas that have functions such as language, sensation, or vision, the patient must actively participate. If a current causes a patient who is awake to stop speaking or to speak in an unintelligible manner, then that area most likely controls language function. Similarly, if a patient reports that a current causes him or her to feel tingling or numbness, the surgeon has discovered a sensory area.

To find out if a particular brain location is contributing to a patient's seizures, it can be useful to activate it using a weak electrical current to observe whether the current triggers a seizure. Even though the current is not painful and cannot be felt by the patient, it interferes with how the area normally functions. Once the current stops, that part of the brain resumes its usual activity

The length of the mapping procedure depends on how much brain tissue is targeted for surgery, how many locations need to be tested, and what kind of functions are expected to reside in those areas. Mapping may take anywhere from one hour to several hours. Cortical mapping has few risks, with the main risk being that a seizure is accidentally triggered. Because the areas being mapped are usually close to where a patient's seizures ordinarily begin, electrical currents applied in this location can set off a seizure. Physicians pay close attention to the patient's brain waves during the stimulation. If electrical discharges that could build up to a seizure are seen, stimulation is immediately stopped. If a patient does have a seizure, mapping is temporarily stopped until the patient has fully recovered.

There is a relatively small risk of pain during electrical stimulation. Even though the brain itself does not sense the currents, an electrode occasionally makes contact with the membranes surrounding the brain. In situations such as these, the patient may feel pain or a tingling sensation when the current is applied. Since the physician always starts at a low current, these contacts are easily identified and avoided.

Reaching a Decision for Surgery

The tests described in this chapter are those that a patient may have on the way to surgery. Once again, patients are individually assessed by their physicians to determine the specific pre-surgical evaluation tests needed. Therefore, each patient will undergo a different set of examinations. Once the pre-surgical evaluation is complete, the patient's case will be presented at a multidisciplinary conference (MDC), where all of the information about the patient, including any preoperative examinations performed, is presented to a group of neurologists, neurosurgeons, neuropsychologists, psychiatrists, and sometimes imaging specialists. Together, these physicians will discuss the patient and reach a decision regarding the type of surgery that is most likely to help. In some centers or hospitals, the decision is made in smaller groups or between the neurosurgeon and the neurologist. Following the MDC, the neurologist will meet with the patient and/or family, inform the patient of the decision reached at the conference, and schedule a consult with the neurosurgeon.

It is critical for physicians to be as thorough as possible when evaluating patients for surgery. Sometimes, it may seem as though too many tests are being performed, but it is necessary to the success of the surgery to have as much information as possible. Surgery is usually a one-time opportunity for becoming seizure-free; it is very rare for a second attempt to be made. Therefore, every precaution must be taken to ensure that the seizure focus is well localized and that the surgery planning is done in such a way that it minimizes any postoperative deficits. In the next chapter, the specific types of epilepsy surgery and their particular applications will be explained in detail.

CHAPTER FOUR
TYPES OF EPILEPSY SURGERY

- Epilepsy surgery does not guarantee complete seizure freedom, but it offers a good chance of total or much better seizure control.
- There are two main types of epilepsy surgery: resective surgery and "disconnection" surgery, a palliative procedure that may help reduce seizure frequency but not offer a cure.
- Resections are performed in single-stage or multistage procedures, depending on how well the seizure focus is identified.
- In a two-stage or multistage procedure, invasive monitoring (intracranial electroencephalogram or EEG) or cortical mapping are performed before and in addition to the resection.
- Temporal lobectomy is the most common type of epilepsy surgery, in which a portion of the dysfunctional temporal lobe is removed to provide the patient complete seizure control.
- Certain special surgeries using other epilepsy surgery techniques may be performed in certain cases depending upon the individual and his or her specific type of epilepsy.
- For those who are viable candidates, epilepsy surgery is considered by far the most effective and comprehensive solution to offering patients a seizure-free life.

Once the pre-surgical evaluation is complete and a decision has been made at a multidisciplinary conference for the best surgery option for the patient, the patient will meet with his or her neurologist. The neurologist will review any test results and explain the consensus reached by the physicians group. Then, the patient will meet with the epilepsy surgeon to review the recommended surgical treatment, the cause for that specific recommendation, the chance of success and subsequent benefits, and the risks of complications or undesired outcome with surgery. Although the potential benefit of surgery always exceeds the current unacceptable condition of intractable seizures, the patient and his or her family must consider the risk of surgery as compared to the risks and quality of life with uncontrolled seizures. Such careful consideration is warranted since sometimes there is more than one surgical option offered. Outcome and associated surgical risks will differ depending on the options. In every case, complete control of seizures cannot be guaranteed, although in the best cases there is a greater than 90 percent chance for complete control.

There are two main types of brain surgery for epilepsy. The first, and by far the most common, is called *resection*, or *resective surgery*. In this type, the surgeon removes the area of the brain that causes the patient's seizures.

The aims of resective surgery are to maximize seizure control and improve quality of life, with the ultimate goal of rendering a patient seizure-free. In a substantial number of patients, resective surgery can mean a cure. The second, less common type of epilepsy surgery interrupts the nerve pathways that allow seizures impulses to spread. The term "disconnection" is sometimes used to describe this type of procedure. A disconnection may be helpful when seizures begin in areas that are too important to the individual's functioning to remove or there are multiple areas causing seizures. Disconnection procedures are palliative (from Latin *palliare*, "to cloak") procedures—they can reduce seizure number, frequency, and severity, but they do not offer a cure. Some of the disconnection procedures are explained in the "Special Surgeries" portion of this chapter. Last, electrical stimulation is sometimes attempted to reduce seizure activity. The *vagus nerve stimulator* and the *response nerve stimulator* are described in detail in Chapter 5.

Resective Surgery

Resective surgery, in which the brain area that causes the seizures is removed, is performed in cases of partial, or focal onset, epilepsy. Patients with partial epilepsy that secondarily generalizes may also be candidates for this type of surgery, as long as the focus of their seizures can be localized. Patients often imagine that the area that causes seizures is tiny. In almost all cases, however, the area is larger. The size of the area of brain tissue to be removed during a resection may be different for each individual. It depends on many variables including the cause, location, and type of epilepsy.

When a localized (focal) area of the brain is found to be the cause of the seizures, it may be possible to remove this tissue and eliminate the seizures completely. However, this area of the brain must be dispensable. In other words, the tissue to be removed should not be one of the critical areas that are needed for movement, sensation, language, or vision. Removal of these important areas of the brain can lead to permanent impairments in the patient's functioning. Fortunately, other brain functions such as personality, intelligence, and the senses of taste and hearing are spread over large areas of brain tissue. Also, the area of the brain that routinely manifests the seizure onset is so abnormal that it does not harbor any useful function, so it is usually safe to resect. As a result, small focal resections of the seizure-onset focus are not likely to cause major deficits in those brain functions. Resections can be performed in *single-stage*, *two-stage*, or *multistage procedures*, depending upon how well the seizure focus has been identified at the time of the surgery. If the focus of the seizure was identified precisely using any of the noninvasive pre-surgical examinations (i.e., magnetic resonance imaging [MRI], video EEG), the neurosurgeon will perform the resection surgery in one stage, or *single-stage*. If, however, a patient's focus cannot be accurately identified using noninvasive techniques, or the focus is located too close to a part of the brain controlling vital functioning, a *two-stage* or *multistage* procedure may be necessary.

In a two-stage procedure, the neurosurgeon will first perform surgery to insert invasive electrodes. These electrodes will either be used for intracranial EEG (Chapter 3), to capture a seizure and localize the focus, or for cortical mapping (Chapter 3), to map the areas of the brain that control important functions that cannot be removed. When enough seizures are captured to accurately define the onset and functional mapping (if needed), is finished, the neurosurgeon will then perform the second stage of the procedure and remove the part of the brain identified as responsible for the seizures.

A multistage procedure is much like a two-stage procedure in that it also involves the placement of intracranial electrodes prior to the removal of brain tissue. However, patients who require multistage resections usually have very complicated cases of epilepsy or have multiple foci that must be removed. Thus, multiple periods of invasive monitoring or mapping may be necessary before the surgical procedure is complete and all of the brain tissue responsible for the seizures has been removed.

Single-Stage Procedures

Patients who undergo single-stage resective surgery have a seizure focus that can be precisely localized using noninvasive techniques (i.e., MRI, video EEG, positron emission tomography [PET]). In these cases, the neurosurgeon can perform the resection without having to do any invasive EEG monitoring beforehand. Examples of single-stage procedures are *lesionectomies*, in which lesions such as tumors or vascular malformations are removed; *temporal resections*, in which a part of the temporal lobe is removed; and *extratemporal resections*, in which a part or parts of the frontal, parietal, or occipital lobes are removed. Each one is explained in the following sections.

Lesionectomy

A lesionectomy (*-ectomy*: to remove) is defined as the surgery to remove a brain lesion. Resections often involve brain surface areas that are found, through testing such as MRI, computed tomography (CT), or PET, to contain physically abnormal tissue. Abnormalities, or lesions, can include scar tissue, benign or malignant tumors, blood vessel malformations, congenital brain malformations, areas of focal atrophy, and other abnormalities. Small lesions are identified as the cause of recurrent seizures in up to 25 percent of epilepsy patients. Modern brain imaging techniques that more accurately detect abnormal anatomic or physiological brain function permit better identification of patients who would benefit from single-stage surgery. Such patients have a 90 percent chance for complete seizure control.

Ideally, the lesionectomy procedure involves the removal of the entire lesion visible on MRI or at time of surgery. However, the presence of nearby critical brain areas, blood vessels, and numerous other factors may limit the size of the resection that can be safely performed. The surgical success rate for patients becoming seizure-free is much higher when a structural brain abnormality is present, as opposed to when there is no well-defined structural brain lesion. This is because the epileptic brain tissue associated with a lesion is typically localized within or adjacent to the lesion, and, if present since birth or early childhood, then reorganization of brain function to more distant areas during development permits safe resection.

MRI and other imaging techniques may not find a visible anatomic abnormality causing seizures. In these situations, EEG recordings, PET scans, and functional MRI (fMRI) are used to show the area of functional abnormality in the brain where the seizures are originating. In other words, if there is no anatomic abnormality then physiologic localization alone must define the resection target, and the techniques of neurosurgery are geared to anatomic resection. Limitations still include the location of the lesion, if the area responsible for seizures is adjacent to or within critical areas of the cortex, and other factors.

Temporal Lobe Resections

If a patient's seizures originate in the temporal lobes, a temporal resection, in which a portion of the temporal lobe is removed, may be performed. Temporal lobe resection is the most common type of epilepsy surgery. Often people use the term temporal lobectomy as synonymous for temporal lobe resection. However, lobectomy means removal of the entire temporal lobe, which is seldom done. Thus, when we discuss or you read about this type of epilepsy surgery, it often refers to temporal lobe resection and not lobectomy.

The temporal lobes are important in memory and emotion. In addition, the upper and back part of one dominant temporal lobe is vital for language comprehension. This "language-dominant" temporal lobe is on the left in nearly all right-handed individuals and in about half of left-handed individuals. Preoperative tests, such as the Wada, assess the potential impact of surgery on memory or language functions by identifying a patient's "language-dominant" temporal lobe, as well as the temporal lobe that controls the majority of memory functioning. During surgery, the surgeon can then avoid those parts of the temporal lobe that are vital to the individual patient's language and memory. In fact, many patients with temporal lobe epilepsy have problems with their verbal or visual-spatial short-term memory even before surgery. This is because this part of their brain, in which seizures are originating, is already functioning improperly, if at all. It is for this reason that epileptogenic brain tissue can be safely removed.

In most cases of temporal resection, a small portion of the brain tissue, the *hippocampus*, is removed, measuring approximately 2 inches in length by 1 inch wide. In general, for a temporal resection, a smaller amount of tissue would be removed from the left hemisphere than from the right hemisphere. This is done to avoid the area in the left temporal lobe that is critical for language comprehension in most individuals.

For patients with epilepsy in whom seizures appear to arise in the deep (mesial) area of the temporal lobe, which includes the hippocampus and adjacent areas, partial removal of the mesial temporal lobe is performed. In this case, a removal of the front (anterior) portion of the temporal lobe is often the first step of the surgery. In this surgery, the surgeon may remove the lobe to a certain distance back from the tip. The next step is for the surgeon to remove the inner (mesial) area of the lobe that contains deeper brain structures known as the *hippocampus*, the *amygdala*, and other adjacent structures (Fig. 13, pg. 60).

These brain structures play an important role in the origin and/or spread of the majority of temporal lobe seizures. Some surgeons remove these mesial tissues as a whole unit, while others remove them piece-by-piece. The advantage of removing the tissue as one piece is that it can be better characterized by the pathologist and therefore confirm the preoperative clinical data to provide a better prediction of prognosis following the surgery.

At a few epilepsy centers, surgeons may prefer to remove only the mesial structures. This variation of mesial temporal lobe surgery is called an *amygdalohippocampectomy*, and it is often a more difficult surgery to perform. It is done with the belief that it may minimize the chance of memory impairment that can occur with temporal lobe resections (Fig. 14, pg. 61). However, many studies suggest that several things predict a low risk of memory impairment with temporal lobe resections. These include the early onset of epilepsy and surgery performed on the side of the brain opposite to the language-dominant temporal lobe.

Personality, mood, and overall behavior are hardly ever disrupted or changed by temporal lobectomy. Part of the explanation is that many brain areas perform similar functions, and so the parts of the brain that control personality, mood, and behavior are located not only in the temporal lobe, but are also spread throughout the brain. Additionally, for people with uncontrolled seizures, the area from which seizures arise can fail to perform the functions normally served by that area, as well as impair function in other normal brain areas. Removal of these areas may actually improve memory and other cognitive functions in some patients post-surgery.

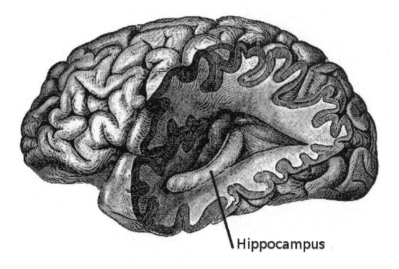

Hippocampus

Figure 13: Location of hippocampus.
(Henry Vandyke Carter [Public Domain]/Wikimedia Commons)

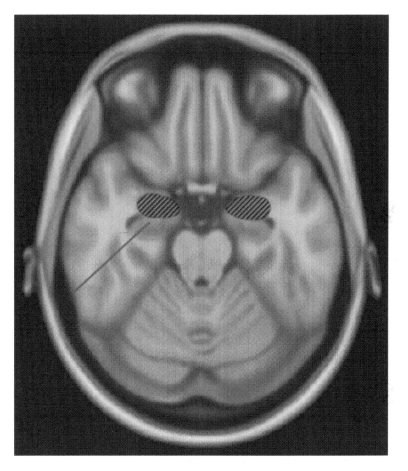

Figure 14: Location of the amygdalae.
(Woutergroen (Own work) [Public domain]/Wikimedia Commons)

Extratemporal Lobe Resections

Extratemporal lobe resections constitute about 30 to 40 percent of the surgical procedures for epilepsy. However, as we advance in our understanding of these more difficult epilepsy disorders, the number of extratemporal epilepsy surgery cases is increasing. In the majority of the cases, this surgery involves the frontal lobe, but it can in certain cases involve the removal of brain tissue from the parietal and/or occipital lobes as well.

The frontal lobes comprise approximately one-third of the cerebral hemisphere. Partial seizures often arise in the frontal lobes. The back part of the frontal lobes (primary motor cortex) controls movement and cannot be removed without causing severe weakness in muscles on the opposite side. In front of the primary motor cortex is the motor association cortex. This area links the primary motor cortex with other brain areas. The motor association cortex can be removed without causing weakness. However, it can be challenging to localize a frontal lobe seizure focus. The large size of the frontal lobe and the relation of some blood vessels make it difficult to record electrical activity from all regions.

Surgery on the parietal or occipital lobes, located in the back of the brain, is most often done when a structural abnormality is identified on the CT or MRI scan (lesionectomy). However, invasive electrode recordings (performed during two-stage or multistage resections) may reveal or confirm that seizures are coming from the parietal or occipital lobes (Fig. 15, pg. 63). The successes and risks of parietal and occipital lobectomies are similar to those of frontal lobectomy. The risk of limb weakness is lower, whereas the risk of impairing touch, sensation, or vision is greater. On the dominant (usually left) side, the parietal lobe is important for language and skilled motor actions. On the nondominant (usually right) side, the parietal lobe is important for spatial perception and ability to focus attention toward the left side of space. The occipital lobes are essential for vision. The left occipital lobe receives information about vision in the right half of space and vice versa.

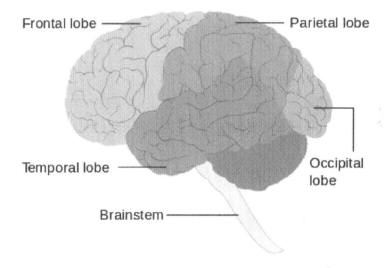

Figure 15: Structure of one brain hemisphere.
(Cancer Research UK/Wikimedia Commons)

Two-Stage Procedures

Although many epilepsy surgeries can be carried out in one stage, a good number of patients require a two-stage procedure in which invasive monitoring (intracranial EEG) or cortical mapping are performed prior and in addition to the resection. The conditions under which two-stage procedures are performed vary widely among epilepsy centers in the United States and around the world. In some epilepsy centers, invasive monitoring is almost always performed prior to surgery, whereas, at other centers, only very rarely is intracranial EEG utilized. The decision to use or not use invasive monitoring and/or cortical mapping is a very complex one and depends upon the center's experience with different technologies, the surgeon's experience and expertise, and other factors.

Patients in which the seizure focus cannot be well-localized using noninvasive techniques often require intracranial EEG. While video EEG utilizes only 16 electrodes and records brain electrical activity from the scalp, intracranial EEG records electrical activity directly from the surface of the brain with a grid or strip of electrodes, which is placed directly on the surface of the brain. Also, depth electrodes that transect or penetrate the brain to sample deep regions out of reach of the surface electrodes may also be used. Over the past decade, we have realized that implanting a greater number of electrodes has improved our characterization of the seizure onset regions, and understanding the complexity of how the seizure manifests and electrically spreads has permitted safer resections with improved seizure control. It is not uncommon to implant more than 50 to 200 individual electrodes contacts (Fig. 16, pg. 66). When a patient has a seizure with intracranial electrodes recording electrical activity, it is possible to obtain a much more precise localization of the seizure focus. The electrodes also show how the seizure spreads and defines the physiological network that is necessary to disrupt with surgery for achieving safer and better surgical seizure control. In addition to intracranial EEG, cortical mapping may sometimes be part of a two-stage resection procedure. Patients who require cortical mapping have seizure origins that appear close to areas of the brain that control vital functions such as movement and language. Using small electrical currents to stimulate specific areas of brain tissue can allow the surgical team to pinpoint those areas that should be avoided during the resection.

For patients undergoing temporal lobe epilepsy resections, it is sometimes necessary to utilize invasive monitoring and/or cortical mapping. If the patient's seizures involve more than the mesial structures (amygdala, hippocampus, etc.), invasive monitoring is sometimes used to define the extent of cortical (surface brain tissue) area that is involved in the seizures and needs to be removed. For patients undergoing a temporal lobectomy on the side of the brain that is language dominant, cortical mapping may be more often utilized. The neurosurgeon must be sure that he or she removes all of the brain tissue causing the seizures while leaving intact the area that controls language. For these procedures, the neurosurgeon first identifies the area of the temporal lobe that controls language. Next, he or she removes the temporal lobe from the tip back as far as possible without damaging any vital tissue.

Some patients who suffer from epilepsy-causing lesions also require invasive monitoring. If the seizures have been present for many years, a considerable area around the lesion may also be involved in the spread of the seizures. With each seizure, over time, the interconnected brain regions become *entrained*, or learn, to be more epileptogenic. This is thought to be the reason why seizures generally worsen over time and require resecting more brain tissue for control. Also, since the normal function of the brain becomes compromised, as it becomes part of the epileptogenic network, some patients experience cognitive decline over time due to uncontrolled epilepsy. This brain tissue may be functioning improperly or not at all. In these cases, invasive monitoring may be necessary to identify how much of the area around the lesion needs to be removed to achieve seizure control.

Unless there is a well-defined, visible lesion, extratemporal lobectomies are almost always guided by localization from invasive electrodes and, if necessary, detailed cortical functional mapping. The large size of the frontal lobe makes it difficult to localize seizure origins without more precise intracranial studies, and the importance of extratemporal tissue for fine motor, language, and visual functioning requires the resections performed in these lobes to be extremely exact. While many temporal lobectomies may look alike, extratemporal resections are different for each individual. They depend upon the seizure onset focus, the type of seizure or syndrome, and functional mapping that defines the safe resection boundary so that essential functions may be kept intact.

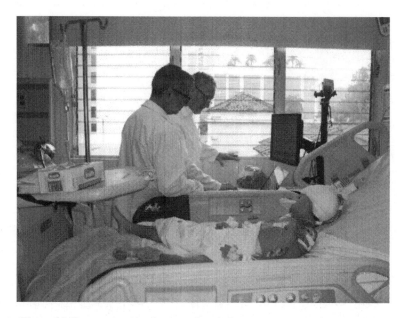

Figure 16: Doctors monitoring a patient in between a two-stage procedure.
(Dr. Ruben Kuzniecky/NYU)

Multistage Procedures

In rare cases, patients undergoing epilepsy surgery require a multistage procedure. For these patients, multiple periods of invasive monitoring, cortical mapping, and even multiple resections, may be performed. An individual who suffers from partial epilepsy with two seizure foci might need to undergo invasive monitoring to identify one seizure focus, the resection to remove that brain tissue, another period of invasive monitoring to identify the other seizure focus, and one last resection to remove that abnormal area. Likewise, if a patient has two seizure foci that are located close to areas controlling vital functions, two separate periods of cortical mapping might be called for. In general, the patients who require a multistage resection procedure are complex in nature.

Special Surgeries

In addition to resection procedures, many other epilepsy surgery techniques are in practice to help patients achieve a greater degree of seizure control. These surgeries are performed only in certain cases that depend upon the individual and his or her specific type of epilepsy. The procedures include *corpus callosotomy*, *hemispherectomy* and variants, *multiple subpial transections* (MSTs), and the specific surgeries to treat hypothalamic hamartoma (HH), cortical dysplasia (CD), tuberous sclerosis complex (TSC), and, finally, stereotactic procedures.

In addition to resection procedures, many other epilepsy surgery techniques are in practice to help patients achieve a greater degree of seizure control. These surgeries are performed only in certain cases that depend upon the individual and his or her specific type of epilepsy. The procedures include *corpus callosotomy*, *hemispherectomy* and variants, *multiple subpial transections* (MSTs), and the specific surgeries to treat hypothalamic hamartoma (HH), cortical dysplasia (CD), tuberous sclerosis complex (TSC), and, finally, stereotactic procedures.

Corpus Callosotomy

Corpus callosotomy (or corpus callosum transection) is a surgical procedure that interferes with the electrical spread of a seizure between the two hemispheres (halves) of the brain. The corpus callosum is a bundle of fibers that connect the right and left hemispheres of the brain to one another. The corpus callosum also ensures that the two halves of the brain communicate

(Fig. 17, pg. 70). When the brain cells (neurons) on one side of the brain transmit electrical signals to the other side, they travel through the fibers that make up the corpus callosum. During a corpus callosotomy, a surgeon divides some portions of, or the entire, corpus callosum. Unlike a resection, a corpus callosotomy does not involve the removal of brain tissue.

In generalized seizures, the fibers of the corpus callosum allow epileptic electrical discharges to rapidly spread throughout the brain. For some patients with severe generalized epilepsy, or multifocal partial epilepsy that generalizes extremely quickly, this rapid spread of epileptic activity can be dangerous. Patients with tonic seizures (seizures that cause sudden body stiffening), atonic seizures (seizures that cause sudden loss of muscle strength), and generalized tonic-clonic seizures (seizures that cause convulsions), often fall as a result of their seizure. In fact, tonic and atonic seizures are also referred to as "drop attacks." These falls can come without warning and may cause serious injuries. Some patients, such as those who have Lennox-Gastaut syndrome, suffer from neurological impairment in the form of mental retardation in addition to a large number of seizures that include "drop attacks." For these patients, when other treatments have failed to reduce the number and severity of seizures, corpus callosotomy can be a viable option. A callosotomy procedure interrupts the neural pathways that cause the rapid generalization of "drop attacks" and convulsions.

Corpus callosotomy was first performed as a treatment for epilepsy in 1939. It was based on the observation of a patient whose generalized seizures improved as a tumor involving the corpus callosum grew larger. There was little interest in callosotomy until the 1960s, when a neurosurgeon published findings on the clinical and neuropsychological outcome of the surgery. Since then, many patients have undergone corpus callosotomy, and the procedure has been modified to produce the best results with the least risk of neurological deficits post-surgery. The technique now involves an initial incision in the scalp at the top of the head. The surgeon then separates the two hemispheres of the brain. Looking into the fissure between the two hemispheres, the surgeon can see the corpus callosum. In patients who do not have severe neurological handicaps before the surgery, the corpus callosum is cut beginning at the front (anterior) end. The cut often extends 50–75 percent toward the back end. Usually, the entire callosum is not cut in order to minimize neurological disconnection symptoms such as inability to read, left arm and leg clumsiness resembling weakness, and inability to name things felt only with the left hand. In some patients with severe pre-existing disabilities, such as severe mental retardation and inability to read, the entire corpus callosum may be cut.

The corpus callosotomy is a palliative surgical procedure—it can reduce but almost never completely eliminate a patient's seizures. The results of the corpus callosotomy can depend on the age of the patient, but, in general, this procedure has a success rate of approximately 50 percent reduction of convulsive and tonic/atonic seizures with a range of 25–70 percent reduction.

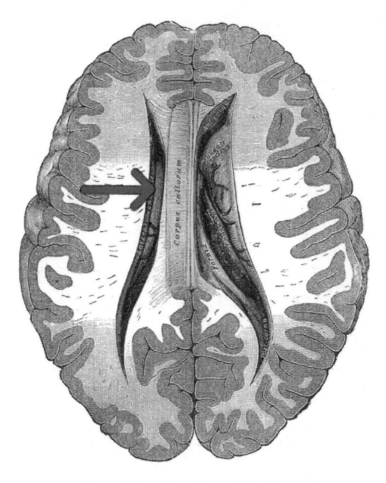

Figure 17: Location of the corpus callosum.
(Henry Vandyke Carter [Public domain]/Wikimedia Commons)

Hemispherectomy and Variants

Hemispherectomy (*hemisphere* = half brain; *ectomy* = removal) is a surgical procedure that originally involved the removal of one entire hemisphere of the brain. Now, it usually involves disconnecting one hemisphere from the rest of the brain, with removal of only a limited area. It is a procedure that is only considered in a small subset of patients with severe epilepsy. Only those individuals who suffer from severe epilepsy in which seizures arise from only one side of the brain and whose brain function in that hemisphere is very impaired are considered candidates. This small percentage of patients has epilepsy that is usually related to a physical condition in one hemisphere of the brain that has been present since birth or early childhood. Examples of these brain disorders that can cause medically refractory seizures at birth are malformations of the cortex, strokes occurring before or just after birth, congenital hemiplegia, chronic encephalitis or Rasmussen's syndrome (a progressive disorder that can lead to severe neurological and intellectual impairment), congenital hemimegalencephaly (a condition in which there is an abnormally large, heavy, and usually malfunctioning brain), and some forms of Sturge-Weber syndrome (a disease present at birth that is caused by malformed blood vessels and may cause neurological abnormalities). Before surgery, patients considered for hemispherectomy typically have weakness and sometimes loss of vision on the opposite side from which the seizures originate. Therefore, the side of the brain that will be disconnected functions very poorly, and the functions of the intact side are being compromised by seizures.

In the past, the dysfunctional hemisphere was removed entirely during a hemispherectomy. However, this sometimes led to long-term complications that could be dangerous to the patient. Therefore, the surgery was modified in the late 1970s, and the procedure performed today is known as *functional hemispherectomy*. Functional hemispherectomy involves separating the upper lobes of the hemisphere from the deep (central) core of the brain and from the opposite hemisphere. This upper separated hemisphere is left in place, connected to its blood vessels, but all the white matter bundles of neurons that pass up and down on that side, and the corpus callosum, are severed. Functional hemispherectomy avoids the possible complications of *hemosiderosis* (an iron overload disorder), *hydrocephalus* (an enlargement of the head caused by an abnormal buildup of cerebrospinal fluid in the brain), and even recurrence of seizures.

Hemispherectomies aim to stop seizures entirely, and this is often achievable in many patients. Hemispherectomies also aim to reverse intellectual and functional decline and, in some cases, to prevent death from *status epilepticus* (a life-threatening condition in which the brain is in a state of persistent seizure). The success rate of hemispherectomies is usually 80–90 percent seizure freedom or significant improvement.

If hemispherectomy is performed on young children as opposed to older patients, the intact hemisphere may make up partly for the loss of brain tissue on the other side. Generally, the more severe the hemiparesis (one-sided weakness) before surgery, the less likely that the patient will have significant weakening of that side post-surgery. Patients who undergo a hemispherectomy will have impaired movement and sensation in the hand, forearm, foot, and leg on the side opposite the operation. The degree of impairment varies from patient to patient. Controlled movements are possible in the upper arm and thigh, thus permitting the individual to walk and use the weak upper limb as a "helper." Physical therapy is often necessary after hemispherectomy surgery.

Multiple Subpial Transections

Multiple subpial transection is an epilepsy surgery procedure that was pioneered as an alternative to the removal of brain tissue. It is used to reduce the frequency and severity of partial seizures originating in areas of the brain that cannot be safely removed. For example, if a seizure focus were located in an area that is critical for language functioning, the removal of this area would devastate the patient's language abilities. Similarly, if the seizure focus is in the area of the brain controlling primary motor functions, complete removal would cause permanent weakness. The operation involves a series of shallow cuts (transections) into the cerebral cortex. The transections are made only as deep as the gray matter, approximately a quarter of an inch into the brain. The transections are made parallel to each other and perpendicular to the long axis of an out-folding (*gyrus*) of the brain. The cuts are thought to selectively interrupt fibers that connect neighboring parts of the brain.

How MST reduces the number of seizures is not fully known, but it is thought to be related to the disconnection of nerve fibers that run horizontally across the cortex, thereby limiting the spread of epileptic electrical discharges. Since the functional units of the cortex are organized perpendicular to the brain's surface extending to the deeper layers, the micro transections of the cortex separate the units without compromising them and still function. This deters the spread of signals between the units without interrupting their function. MST can be performed as the sole surgical procedure, or it can be accompanied by focal cortical resection. Most neurosurgeons believe the best results are achieved when MSTs are combined with resection.

The MST technique was first described in a large group of patients in 1989. Since then, physicians have reported good reductions of seizures with little or no neurological deficits post-surgery. Multiple subpial transections can help reduce and, in some cases, even eliminate seizures arising from vital functional cortical areas. Some patients with frontal and temporal lobe epilepsy are candidates for MST. The procedure can also be successful in Landau-Kleffner syndrome (a disorder in which language problems occur in a child whose language was previously developing normally), Rasmussen syndrome, and in patients with scars or birth malformations of brain cortex that have been determined to contain functional regions.

Although the initial short-term results of MST were encouraging, the long-term results may not be so promising. The number of procedures has fallen in the past decade because the results have been less than desired. In general, there is a 30–40 percent chance of worthwhile improvement, but in some centers the results have been reported to be better. As stated, one concern with MST is that the epileptic activity that was stopped by the procedure may recur after a period of 2–20 months. This procedure may achieve long-term reduction of seizure activity, but it is not as effective as removal or disconnection of the seizure focus. Although MST is still somewhat controversial, experience with this surgical technique has shown that it is a safe and important option for many patients.

Special Syndromes and Procedures

Certain medical syndromes sometimes lead to the development of epilepsy and seizures in some people. For these patients, seizure medication does not often provide relief from seizures, and epilepsy surgery may be a very good option if they are good candidates. A few examples of these syndromes are listed next.

Hypothalamic Hamartomas

Hypothalamic hamartomas (HH) are rare congenital malformation that occur on the hypothalamus during fetal development and are present at birth. Although the lesions are tumor-like and grow with the brain, they do not spread or become cancerous (Fig. 18, pg. 75).

Symptoms for HH vary greatly in severity and type from patient to patient, but they're apparent during childhood for a large number of patients. *Gelastic* (laughing) seizures and epilepsy are commonly seen in patients with HH, often during infancy. Similar to other epilepsy patients, some with HH-related seizures suffer from developmental delay and cognitive decline, as well as psychiatric symptoms like violent "rage" behavior and precocious puberty. Antiepileptic drugs (AEDs) do not usually control seizures associated with HH, and seizures often worsen over time.

Although HH and epilepsy have been known for more than a century, it was not until the 1990s that investigators discovered that the seizures were arising from the hamartomas. Up until then, EEG studies had always shown abnormalities in different brain regions, indicating that any type of surgery would not be beneficial. In fact, many of these patients had temporal or frontal resections without benefits. In addition, surgeons tried to remove the hamartomas using routine surgical techniques with poor results and complications. Having proved that the lesions themselves were the source of the seizures, several teams developed surgical and nonsurgical approaches with good results and fewer complications. Currently, *gamma knife* may be a good choice for some patients, while *stereotactic radiofrequency* or *laser therapy* may be better for others. Another technique uses an endoscopic approach from the top of the brain through the corpus callosum and down into the hypothalamus (see Figure on next page) with removal of the abnormal tissue. Good long-term seizure control has been reported for all of these techniques, with relatively low complications. However, not all patients are seizure free and many need medications long-term.

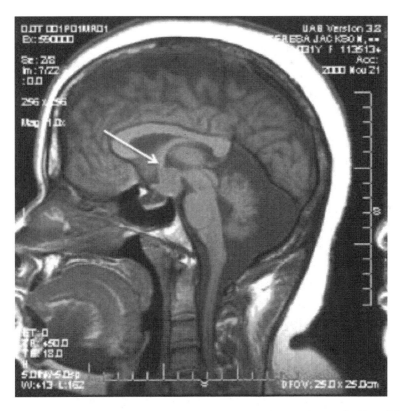

Figure 18: MRI scan scan of a patient with hypothalamic hamartoma (indicated by arrow). These benign lesions cause significant seizures and behavioral problems. Targeted surgery may help alleviate symptoms.
(Dr. Ruben Kuzniecky/NYU)

Tuberous Sclerosis

Tuberous sclerosis, also called *tuberous sclerosis complex* (TSC), is a rare genetic disease that causes benign tumors to grow in the brain and on other vital organs, such as the kidneys, heart, eyes, lungs, and skin (Fig. 19, pg. 77). Like with HH, patients with TSC very often suffer from seizures and behavioral issues. As a result, a majority of TSC patients have developmental delays that vary in severity by individual.

The surgical approach in TS patients is divided in two groups. First, there are TS patients who have a single area causing seizures even though the brain has many tubers. If pre-surgical testing shows a single tuber or brain region as the source of focal seizures, the patient maybe a good candidate for surgery, and removal of a single tuber or tuber area may result in good surgical outcome. The other group, which is unfortunately more common, consists of those patients who have multiple areas of seizures corresponding to multiple brain tubers. In these patients, surgery can be done, but it requires complex intracranial EEG studies and surgeries.

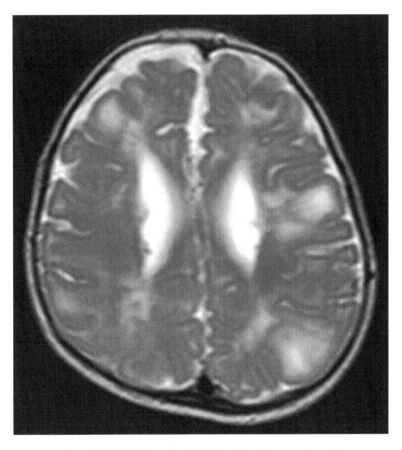

Figure 19: MRI of patient's brain with tuberous sclerosis.
Note the many abnormal areas throughout the brain.
(Hellerhoff (Own work) [CC BY-SA 3.0]/ Wikimedia Commons)

Focal Cortical Dysplasia

Focal cortical dysplasia (FCD) is a congenital abnormality of brain development that occurs when an area of the brain does not form properly. It is the most common cause of medically refractory epilepsy in children and also a very common cause for intractable seizures in adults. There are three types of FCD, all of which range in severity in relation to the brain functions they disrupt and the seizures the patients experience.

Most often in patients with FCD present with focal epilepsy. MRI can detect certain types of FCD but the resolution is not good enough for those with subtle lesions. If the MRI and EEG are concordant and the FCD is at a distance from critical brain areas, complete resection may provide cure or major improvement. If the lesions are close to critical brain regions and total resection is not feasible, the results maybe not be so beneficial. Most patients with FCD require implantation of intracranial EEGs to map and locate the seizure focus. Studies over the past decades have shown a correlation between good outcome and total lesion resection.

Stereotactic Procedures

Stereotactic techniques refer to surgery using computer navigation and guidance devices that permit the neurosurgeon to implant electrodes or probes, or direct the surgical approach from the brain surface to deeper regions with less invasive and more accurate trajectories. Modern neurosurgery routinely uses computer navigation and stereotactic guidance that permits less invasive, more accurate, and safer surgery. Similar to a GPS system that directs an automobile driver from one location to another by integrating the road map to where the driver is at any moment, the stereotactic methods direct the surgeon by integrating the actual surgical technique to the unique anatomy of the patient as defined by the patient's MRI.

Laser Ablation

The Visualase MRI-guided laser ablation technology is one example of this new method in neurosurgery. Guided by MRI images, the Visualase delivers precise laser energy to the target area using a laser applicator, which ultimately destroys the targeted tissue. Because it is minimally invasive compared to traditional open procedures, fewer sutures are needed, and there is often little to no hair removal at the surgical site. In one major advantage over pure radiofrequency ablation that uses heat, the Visualase system uses MRI temperature images to monitor the amount of tissue being targeted. This offers improved accuracy over radiofrequency and direct observation of the target during the procedure.

Although promising, this is a new technique that, although applied already to general neurosurgery, it is still in its infancy for epilepsy. There are several potential advantages such as better targeting, less invasiveness than open cranial surgery, lower cost, possible less memory dysfunction, and shorter hospital stay. Few studies with enough long-term follow-up are available to assess how much better this technique is than open surgery. A recent study reported that following targeted lesion of the hippocampus for mesial temporal epilepsy, 8 of 15 patients (53 percent) and 4 of 11 patients (36 percent) were seizure-free after 6 months. Furthermore, four patients had an anterior temporal lobectomy (ATL) after the laser therapy because of recurrent seizures. One patient had significant complications. Other studies have also reported similar results.

It is clear that MRI-guided stereotactic laser therapy is an alternative to ATL in patients with medically intractable temporal lobe epilepsy. However, careful assessment is needed to determine whether the reduced odds of seizure freedom are worth the reduction in risk, discomfort, and recovery time. Larger studies are needed to confirm early experience.

Radiosurgery

Radiosurgery refers to the method of focusing a large number of thin beams of radiation onto a small volume of brain tissue, targeting the brain tissue using stereotactic methods similar to surgical navigation. Only where the beams are focused does the radiation dose exceed the ability of the exposed brain to recover from the harmful effects of radiation. So only brain tissue in the focal point of the many beams of radiation dies, and the remainder of the brain, though receiving the radiation as the beams travel through it, recovers without permanent injury. With this technique, deep-seated regions of the brain can be destroyed with radiation without opening the skull and performing conventional surgery. This is why radiosurgery is sometimes referred to as "brain surgery without a knife" or noninvasive surgery. While this technique can be useful for small tumors or vascular malformations, it has not gained acceptance in epilepsy surgery for several reasons. The most important problem is that the radiated brain tissue becomes necrotic after it dies, causing swelling and inflammation of the surrounding tissue, further resulting in dysfunction of the adjacent brain.

For about one in four patients receiving radiotherapy for epilepsy, the inflammation is so severe that conventional surgery must be performed to remove the necrotic brain. Routinely, the patient's seizures worsen for up to

12 months following radiosurgery before any reduction in seizures is appreciated. Frequent MRI scans are required to monitor the effects of the radiation for a year or more. And only patients who are candidates for single-stage epilepsy surgery can be offered radiosurgery since only those patients have a well-defined lesion—an absolute requirement for the radiosurgery. Therefore, only patients with medially intractable epilepsy and mesial temporal sclerosis are candidates for radiosurgery.

Since a single-stage surgery for this form of epilepsy provides immediate control of the seizures, patients do not need multiple MRI follow-ups, and only 1 percent of cases require reoperation (rather than the 25 percent for complications related to the therapy). Almost all epilepsy surgeons and epilepsy centers prefer to offer conventional anteromedial temporal lobectomy rather than radiotherapy to their patients. The 70–90 percent complete control rate for conventional surgery has not been routinely duplicated with radiosurgery, further discouraging the use of radiotherapy. The only likely use could be for patients with well-defined temporal lobe epilepsy who refuse to have open cranial surgery.

Risks of Surgery for Epilepsy

In general, craniotomy for epilepsy-related procedures is associated with a 1 percent incidence of significant complication usually due to stroke or bleeding. This results in a permanent brain injury and a neurological disability. Infection occurs in about 3 percent of procedures involving implantation of electrodes for invasive monitoring (i.e., for staged operations). Infection rate is only 1 percent for single-stage procedures. Although infection does not result in a permanent neurological disability, it often requires additional surgical intervention to clean out the infected wound and remove the craniotomy bone plate, producing a skull defect that is repaired some months later after the infection has been cured.

Other risks include anesthesia risks, medication reactions, blood loss requiring transfusion, blood clots in the leg (deep vein thrombosis or DVT) or lungs (pulmonary embolism or PE), pneumonia, urinary tract infection, and any other adverse consequence associated with any major surgery. Usually, these adverse events can be corrected without any long-term consequences. In patients older than 55 years, some of these complications may be more serious, especially DVT that can progress to PE, which can be life-threatening. Death due to surgery is very rare (1/1,000) and much less likely than death as a consequence of uncontrolled epilepsy.

Benefits of Cranial Surgery for Epilepsy

The goal for some cranial procedures is *palliation* or improvement in seizures. However, for most types of epilepsy surgery, the intention is for complete seizure control, without necessarily the complete elimination of the need for medical management. In the best candidates for epilepsy surgery, those who undergo a single-stage temporal lobe resection, complete seizure control is achieved in 70–90 percent of cases. The two-stage procedures achieve at least a 65 percent possibility for complete seizure control outcome. The most difficult cases, typically requiring multistage surgery, offer at most a 50 percent chance for complete control. On the whole, important seizure control is achieved in three out of four patients who undergo epilepsy surgery. It must be understood that reports of seizure control by different epilepsy centers vary since outcome is dependent upon patient selection, the type of seizures being treated, the techniques used by the surgeons, and even by the biases of the referring neurologists and physicians who influence what sort of patient the epilepsy centers receives. There are no standard or accepted criteria for selecting patients for epilepsy surgery, nor for which surgical procedure is necessarily more or less appropriate for the different settings and epilepsy presentations. The largest epilepsy centers usually tend to treat the most difficult patients. However, experience of the surgical multidisciplinary team is the most important ingredient for the safest and best surgical outcomes (see Table 4.1, pg. 82).

Reoperation for Surgical Failure to Control Epilepsy

Epilepsy surgery failures are often reevaluated to determine why the original surgery was not effective. In those patients where reevaluation suggests that further resection or another epilepsy surgery may be useful, further surgery is offered. In patients deemed to be candidates for further surgery, up to one half of them who elect to pursue reoperation will become seizure-free or improve from the second epilepsy surgery, while the other 50 percent may not see much change. The most common reason for failure of the initial surgery is that not enough of the epileptogenic network was resected.

This is not an uncommon reason for failure since the accepted philosophy of surgery is that whenever it is unclear how much brain to remove, less rather than more will be resected. In this way, the primary goal of epilepsy surgery to not produce any important neurological compromise is satisfied. However, reevaluating failures may reveal that residual epileptogenic tissue remains, providing evidence not able to be obtained otherwise that the questionable tissue must be removed.

Table 4.1

Percentage of Patients Achieving Seizure Freedom

After Various Types of Epilepsy Surgery

Type of Surgery	% Patients with Seizure Freedom
Lesionectomy	70–90%
Temporal Lobectomy (Mesial)	70–90%
Temporal Lobectomy (Lateral)	50%
Extratemporal Lobectomy	40–50%
Callosotomy*	50%
Hemispherectomy	80-90%
Reoperation	≤50%

* Callosotomy is a palliative procedure. Fifty percent of patients will have worthwhile improvement.

Summary

Epilepsy surgery today is largely considered the most comprehensive and effective solution to living a seizure-free life. While it is becoming less of a last-resort option for many epilepsy patients, there may be many reasons why someone may not be a good candidate for surgery. Patients for whom resective or disconnection surgery is not a viable option or who don't feel mentally and emotionally prepared for surgery may alternatively consider electrical stimulation therapy, as explained in the next chapter.

CHAPTER FIVE
ELECTRICAL STIMULATION THERAPY
IN EPILEPSY

- Neuromodulation can be a good alternative treatment for patients with treatment-resistant epilepsy who are not considered good candidates for seizure focus resection.

- Therapies like vagus nerve stimulation (VNS) and responsive neurostimulation (RNS) are commonly used today as palliative options for patients with medically refractory epilepsy.

- VNS is extracranial and is implanted in the neck and chest area like a pacemaker. It is thought to work by delivering electrical stimulation to the vagus nerve, the longest of the 12 pairs of cranial nerves originating from the brain. About 30–40 percent of patients with VNS will report a 50 percent reduction in seizure frequency and often a reduction in seizure intensity.

- Directly implanted in the brain, RNS works by delivering electrical impulses to the brain when it detects a change in brainwave activity associated with a seizure pattern. Although this therapy is new and data are limited, more than 50 percent of patients report a 50 percent reduction in seizures with RNS.

- Not yet approved by the U.S. Food and Drug Administration (FDA) for epilepsy treatment, DBS was first used for seizures in the 1970s and is being studied again today. Directly implanted in the brain, it involves placing electrodes into various deep brain areas, which deliver intermittent electrical pulses similar to VNS.

- Although complete seizure control is uncommon with neuromodulation treatments, they can possibly offer a better quality of life by reducing seizure frequency and intensity in in place of or in combination with resective surgery.

Electrical Stimulation (Neuromodulation)

While resective surgery is considered the most effective solution to eliminating seizures for patients with medically refractory epilepsy, it may not be the safest or most viable option for everyone. Alternatively, electrical stimulation, or neuromodulation, is the best treatment for patients with refractory epilepsy who are not considered good candidates for resective surgery due to seizures arising from functional areas of the brain or more than two areas or in patients in whom a resection failed to control seizures. Neuromodulation broadly refers to an emerging number of therapies that primarily involve targeted electrical stimulation of the central nervous system to restore function, influence brain tissue, relieve pain, or control symptoms such as seizures in patients with epilepsy or tremor in patients with Parkinson's disease. Electrical stimulation therapies, such as vagus nerve stimulation (VNS) and responsive neurostimulation (RNS), are used today to help control seizures in patients with epilepsy who do not have acceptable outcomes or control with antiepileptic drugs (AEDs) alone and who are also not candidates for resective surgery. In this chapter, we describe these modes of therapy now available to treat epilepsy, starting with VNS, which has been available since 1997, and RNS, which was recently approved by the U.S. FDA in November 2013.

Vagus Nerve Stimulation

The vagus nerve is the longest of 12 pairs of nerves that originate directly from the brain; these are called *cranial nerves* (all other nerves come off the spinal cord). These cranial nerves conduct electrical impulses and subserve important sensory and motor functions, including vision (optic nerve), hearing (auditory nerve), taste, smell (olfactory nerve), facial movement and sensation, eye movement, head movement, shoulder movement, and mouth and tongue movements. By directing information to and from equally important deep brain regions that connect to and interact with broad regions of the brain, the cranial nerves can influence brain behavior. It is believed that vagus nerve stimulation influences the brain by altering brain activity, which results in electrical desynchronization as observed by electroencephalogram (EEG). In other words, different brain areas are less likely to appear similar or synchronized on EEG. Since a seizure is a *hypersynchronous* (better organized) rhythm on EEG, vagus nerve stimulation makes it less likely for a seizure to occur. Despite this, the exact mechanism by which the VNS works in epilepsy is still unknown after many years of using the device.

The FDA approved VNS in 1997 to help treat medically refractory partial epilepsy for people aged 12 and older. In clinical trials, seizure frequency was reduced by an average of 45 percent, with a 36 percent reduction at 3 to12 months after implantation and a 50 percent reduction of seizures after more than a year of therapy. Approximately 10 percent of patients experience up to a 90 percent decrease in seizures. However, long-term follow-up and clinical experience suggest that seizure reduction is much more variable, with about one-third of the patients benefiting from major reduction in seizure frequency, one-third experiencing no change, and one-third reporting variable or moderate reductions in seizure frequency.

Despite its clinical ability to reduce seizures, it is very important to remember that complete seizure control with VNS is very rare; less than 5 percent of patients report being 100 percent seizure-free. Because it offers partial seizure control, VNS is considered an add-on therapy for epilepsy and is used in conjunction with a medication regimen.

Because cranial surgery has the potential to control seizures completely, VNS is typically not the best or first option for patients who are candidates for cranial surgery. Alternatively, some patients choose to try the less invasive VNS first before opting for cranial surgery. VNS is most often used in the following scenarios:

1. Patients are not candidates for focal resection because the risk of surgery outweighs the benefits. For example, surgery in speech, motor, or visual areas of the brain will cause significant language problems or will result in loss of vision on one side.
2. Patients have generalized epilepsies (those that are diffuse in nature) where focal resections are not likely possible.
3. Patients have multifocal seizures.
4. People underwent cranial surgery but failed to get seizure control and are not candidates for either further resection surgery or RNS.

Unlike with a resection, VNS does not require a brain operation and is often done as an outpatient procedure. The vagus nerve travels from the brain to the rest of the body by going through the neck. Relatively superficial (under the skin of the neck) and large, the vagus nerve can be easily exposed, allowing for a small wire electrode to be wrapped around it (Fig. 20, pg. 87). The VNS device generator (resembling a cardiac pacemaker) contains a battery and is implanted into the chest. The surgeon first makes an incision on the left outer side of the chest and implants the device under the skin. Then a second incision is made in the lower neck and a wire is wrapped around the vagus nerve. The wire is tunneled under the skin, connecting the electrode to the generator. At the end of the procedure, two small scars are left, one on the neck and one on the chest (Fig. 21, pg. 90).

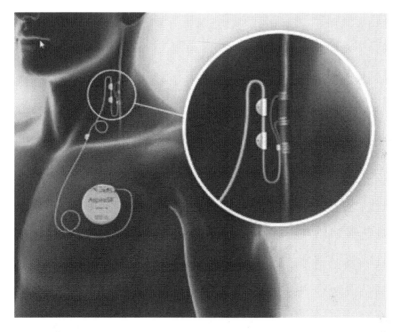

Figure 20: The VNS device consists of a stimulator placed in the chest and wires connected to the vagus nerve in the neck.
(Cyberonics/Livonova Corporation)

The surgical procedure takes less than two hours to perform. VNS implantation is generally very well-tolerated, and the patient will typically go home the same day of the procedure. The most notable risks associated with VNS implantation are infection and injury to the vagus nerve, both of which have a very low occurrence, ranging from about 1 to 5 percent of patients, depending on the center and surgeon's experience. If the vagus nerve is damaged during the surgery, the person may have a permanent change in voice hoarseness. Once the device is turned on, the patient will not feel it operating. Only during the stimulation are possible side effects experienced (tingling, hoarseness, mild discomfort), and they are generally well-tolerated. Transient side effects are common and include hoarseness or a change in voice during the "on" or stimulation period; this is reported by 40–60 percent of patients. Other transient side effects include cough, *paresthesia* (a feeling of numbness, burning, tickling, or "pins and needles"), pain, *dyspnea* (shortness of breath), and headaches.

To optimize seizure control, the healthcare team will adjust the stimulation parameters by communicating with the generator via a small handheld device placed over the generator in the chest well. These adjustments take about 10–15 minutes to do in the outpatient office.

There are many parameters (higher current, shorter duration, faster cycles, etc.) that can be set in the VNS. The most common protocol is to stimulate the nerve for 30 seconds every 5 minutes, but faster protocols are possible. The VNS continuously works on and off 24 hours a day. Another feature is that the patient can also trigger the VNS device to deliver a burst of stimulation outside of the programmed intervals using a magnet placed over the chest and then removed. This feature can be especially useful for people who experience auras that warn them of an impending seizure, possibly allowing for time to stop it from occurring. The same thing can be said about patients who experience convulsive seizures. Family members may be able to activate the VNS with a magnet during a seizure to try to stop or reduce the length or intensity of the convulsive event. However, this rescue maneuver to stop or reduce a seizure is quite variable among patients.

Magnetic resonance imaging (MRI) scans are still safe with VNS implantation as long as the patient wears a head coil. Turning off the device during an MRI scan is also an option.

Battery life of the VNS generator is typically 5–10 years (depending on the settings used), so if the device proves to help control seizures, the battery will need to be replaced with a new one through another outpatient surgery. For this procedure, only the generator is replaced, without the need to replace the electrode.

Unlike medication, which can lose its efficacy to control seizures over time, VNS will actually either improve its ability to control seizures or remain unchanged. Additionally, it can be used in some patients to help reduce the number and dose of anticonvulsant medications, thereby reducing adverse medication side effects.

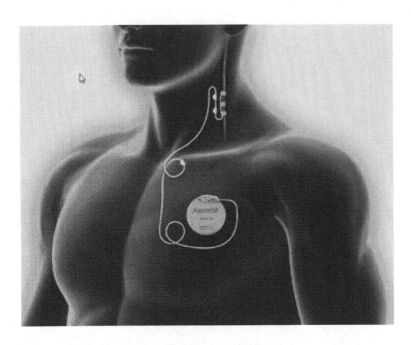

Figure 21: The VNS device implantation requires the surgeon to make two small incisions in the neck and chest.
(Cyberonics/Livonova Corporation)

Results of VNS Therapy

Although VNS was initially approved only for adults and adolescents older than 12 who suffer from partial onset seizures (seizures that begin in one part of the brain), studies have shown that children experience a slightly better outcome with VNS than do adults (55 percent versus 50 percent reduction in seizures, respectively), with patients younger than 6 years seeing up to 60 percent decrease in seizures. Additionally, patients with generalized epilepsy (in which seizures involve the whole brain) have shown to have better results with VNS therapy than those with partial epilepsy (58 percent versus 43 percent reduction in seizures, respectively). Even so, because there is currently a lack of sufficient studies and supportive data studying the efficacy of VNS therapy in both children and in patients with generalized epilepsy, it cannot be said definitively whether they specifically see an increased benefit. However, study findings do suggest that both of these patient groups may find some seizure relief from VNS, though they were initially excluded during the FDA clinical trials.

Although the FDA approved VNS in 1997 as an adjunctive treatment for medically refractory epilepsy, it is still difficult to predict which patients will benefit the most. In a recent large study, investigators tried to address this problem by doing a meta-analysis of published data. These authors performed the first meta-analysis of VNS efficacy in epilepsy, identifying 74 clinical studies with 3,321 patients suffering from intractable epilepsy. These studies included three blinded, randomized controlled trials (Class I evidence); two non-blinded, randomized controlled trials (Class II evidence); 10 prospective studies (Class III evidence); and numerous retrospective studies. After VNS, seizure frequency was reduced by an average of 45 percent, with a 36 percent reduction in seizures at 3–12 months after surgery and a 51 percent reduction after more than 1 year of therapy. At the last follow-up, seizures were reduced by 50 percent or more in approximately 50 percent of the patients, and VNS predicted up to a 50 percent reduction in seizures.

Patients with generalized epilepsy and children benefited significantly from VNS despite their exclusion from initial approval of the device. Furthermore, post-traumatic epilepsy and tuberous sclerosis were positive predictors of a favorable outcome. In conclusion, VNS is an effective and relatively safe adjunctive therapy in patients with medically refractory epilepsy not amenable to resection. However, it is important to recognize that complete seizure freedom is rarely achieved using VNS, and 50 percent of patients do not receive any benefit from therapy.

Responsive Neurostimulation

In 2013, after many years of development and clinical trials, the FDA approved responsive neurostimulation (RNS) to help treat patients who suffer from partial seizures. Operating on a "closed-loop" system, the RNS implant directly stimulates the brain with electric pulses through a battery-powered device (called the *neurostimulator*) implanted in the skull. The stimulator is connected to two EEG wires that are placed on the surface and/or inside of the brain where seizures originate. Unlike the VNS, which delivers intermittent electrical pulses at a programmed schedule, RNS only stimulates the brain when it detects abnormal EEG activity (a seizure).

The stimulator has both a computer that can detect and record a seizure and a stimulator that can deliver electric pulses through the electrodes. Parameters for detection and stimulation are individually set for each patient.

Because the technology is relatively new and takes time to analyze and program, it is unknown whether RNS offers better seizure control than VNS. In fact, no studies are available to date comparing both treatments. The RNS directly targets the brain area causing seizures, while the VNS stimulates the entire brain through the vagus nerve. Between 30 and 40 percent of patients report considerable improvements in seizure severity or frequency. More than 50 percent of patients treated with RNS in the main clinical trial had a 50 percent reduction of seizure frequency lasting up to 80 months. Long-term follow-ups with patients in the study showed that the percentage increased steadily over the first 2–3 years after the RNS device was implanted, reaching up to 55 percent. During the 4-year follow-up period for the initial study patients, 20 percent were seizure-free for periods of 6 months or more. The average reduction in seizure frequency at 12 months after the implant was about 40 percent, increasing to 51 percent at 24 months.

Like VNS therapy, RNS should not be viewed as a cure for epilepsy but rather as a palliative procedure that offers partial relief from seizures, the significance of which cannot be appreciated unless the device is implanted. However, since RNS targets the brain by stimulating it directly (unlike VNS), it has a higher probability for improved seizure control. For this reason, it is best suited for patients who are candidates for focal resection but who cannot have a resection because the brain area responsible for the seizures is likely to cause significant and unacceptable neurologic deficits if resected.

For example, a patient with focal temporal lobe seizures with a Wada test that demonstrates intact memory function may be rendered seizure-free from surgery, but at a cost of significant, unacceptable memory loss. Another indication is for patients who have temporal seizures arising from both temporal lobes. In these patients, surgery in one temporal lobe may only reduce seizures, which may not result in significant improvement in quality of life or acceptable outcome for some patients. Patients with multifocal seizures outside of the temporal lobe and those for whom a resection did not completely eliminate seizures may benefit from RNS targeting the remaining epileptic tissue if the remaining tissue is viable for stimulation. However, since the RNS is relatively new at this point, we are still in the process of understanding what seizure types are the most amenable to RNS therapy and what patients make the best candidates.

Implanting the RNS device requires the doctors to know the approximate area responsible for the patient seizures. The RNS is implanted by intracranial surgery, which usually takes approximately 4–6 hours in an operating room. Typically, the skull is opened by making small holes in the skull bone. Then the electrodes are inserted or placed in the areas targeted for stimulation. Once the electrodes are in place, the *dura* (the tissue that covers the brain) is closed. Next, the neurosurgeon places the stimulation device into the skull by making a small indentation into the skull and connecting the electrodes to the generator. Finally, the scalp is closed, making the entire device and electrodes invisible (Fig. 22, pg. 94). The device is immediately turned on and programmed to capture and record EEG seizure activity without delivering any stimulation. Most patients spend two nights in the hospital after the implantation.

As with any neurosurgery procedure, risks with RNS implantation can include bleeding, infection, direct injury to the brain tissue, stroke, or hemorrhage, which can result in permanent neurological impairment. Most commonly, patients experience headache and mild pain at the implant site for a few days to a couple of weeks. The complication rates have been low in RNS clinical trials, and so far these low rates have been duplicated in clinical practice. Generally, the benefits associated with RNS exceed the risks, and this should be discussed in depth with the neurosurgeon before proceeding with surgery. Patients should also ask the surgeon how many RNS surgeries he or she has performed and his or her complication rate. Patients are also encouraged to get a second opinion.

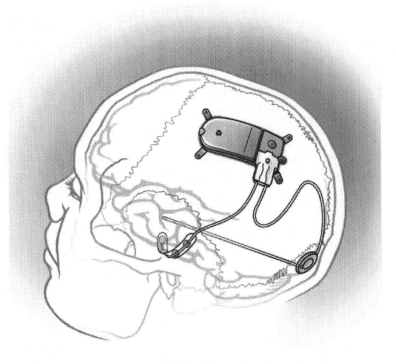

Figure 22: The RNS is connected to electrodes in the brain surface or in the brain tissue.
(Neuropace Corporation)

About 10–14 days following RNS implantation, the patient will meet with his or her surgical and epilepsy care team or clinicians in the outpatient office to check on how the surgical site is healing and determine how many seizures have been recorded. Additionally, the patient will be provided with a laptop computer and a hand-held "wand" that uses radiofrequency (RF) communication to collect data from the neurostimulator. Using a special software program installed on a laptop, the patient holds the wand over the skull where the RNS is located and connects the wand to the computer, thus allowing it to collect all the data from the neurostimulator. These data are then sent remotely from home by the patient to a database called a Patient Data Management System (PDMS), where the patient's doctor can access it to make adjustments to the neurostimulator during future visits (Fig. 23, pg. 97). The RNS device will then be programmed to detect future seizures, and stimulation parameters are set based on the history of seizure frequency and severity. This feature is advantageous because it allows for more targeted treatment for each individual patient based on his or her particular seizure type.

Subsequent appointments will take place 4–6 weeks following surgery and then about every 3 months to continue monitoring of seizures and the treatment. After reviewing the data recorded by the neurostimulator, the epileptologist can make necessary adjustments through a special computer that communicates with the implanted RNS generator at any time. Another useful feature is that additional electrodes can be connected to the stimulator if the original electrode combination fails to target the main epileptogenic areas. This is done by accessing the RNS generator located just under the skin. The skin needs to be opened and the leads disconnected and reconnected during a day surgery or outpatient surgical procedure. Patients do not need to stay overnight in the hospital for this operation.

Although a very small percentage of patients report being able to feel the stimulation, there are little to no side effects directly associated with RNS stimulation except those immediately experienced at the time of the surgery. Furthermore, if the patient feels stimulation, the settings are lowered to alleviate any discomfort or side effects.

Battery life for the neurostimulator is about 2–3.5 years and is dependent on the stimulation settings set by the doctor and the frequency of seizures resulting in stimulation. When the battery gets very low, a minor surgery will be performed to replace the depleted neurostimulator in its secured holder in the skull with a new one. The same EEG leads will usually be reconnected to the new neurostimulator unless they also need to be replaced. This surgery is relatively small, with fewer side effects and risk because the bone is not opened, only the skin. The electrodes are typically left in place and reattached to the new RNS generator.

There is a chance that RNS will not improve seizure frequency or severity. However, in clinical trials, its efficacy has been shown to increase over time, with more than half of patients seeing a 50 percent reduction in seizure frequency after 2 years with the device. As with VNS treatment, RNS shows potential for improving seizure control with less medication for patients with medically refractory focal epilepsy. However, at this time, information and outcome data are limited to predict who the best candidates for RNS implantation are, the type of seizures that respond best to RNS, and the long-term effects on seizures, memory, or other brain functions.

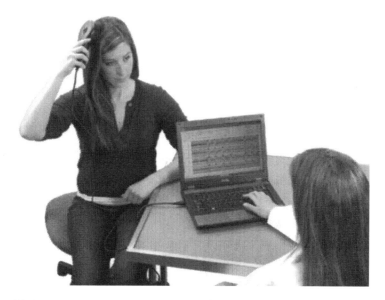

Figure 23: The patient's doctor can make adjustments to the RNS device's settings based on the data collected by the hand-held "wand" and sent to the Patient Data Management System.
(Neuropace Corporation)

Deep Brain Stimulation

Although not yet approved by the FDA for epilepsy therapy, deep brain stimulation (DBS) was first used experimentally to help treat epilepsy in the 1970s, and it is used commonly today to offer symptomatic relief to patients suffering from movement disorders, such as Parkinson's disease and essential tremor, for which it is has FDA approval. DBS therapy is being studied again for epilepsy treatment, and initial studies have shown that people with medically refractory epilepsy have had fewer seizures after DBS of the thalamus. The treatment involves placing electrodes into various deep brain areas and connecting them to a computerized pulse generator that is implanted under the skin below the collarbone. The neurostimulator is programmed to deliver predetermined intermittent electrical stimulation to the brain at settings thought to restore normal brain activity; this works similarly to VNS. Unlike RNS, which senses and responds to seizure activity, DBS sends an electrical signal at regularly determined times and doses regardless of brain activity.

To date, there is not enough evidence to show efficacy of DBS for treating seizures, and experimental trials have demonstrated varying results. For some patients, seizures become much less frequent and severe, while there is little to no effect for others. It can also take up to 2 years for DBS therapy to begin to show an effect.

In the largest clinical trial (Sentinel trial) published in 2010, patients who received DBS implantation in the thalamus after an initial 3-month placebo phase saw a reduction in seizures by 40 percent. In comparison, a control group who had the stimulator device implanted but did not receive any stimulation had a 14.5 percent reduction in seizures. After 13 months of DBS, 41 percent of patients showed fewer seizures, while 43 percent of patients had their seizures reduced by at least 50 percent. After 25 months, 56 percent of patients reported fewer seizures, and 54 percent saw a 50 percent reduction. At 37 months, 67 percent of patients had at least a 50 percent reduction of seizures. Of the 110 patients in the study, 14 (or 12.7 percent) were seizure-free for at least 6 months.

Like VNS and RNS, DBS is not a cure for epilepsy. It is used in conjunction with AEDs to help better control seizures. If the treatment shows efficacy, there is a possibility of reducing medications over time. This is always done slowly and methodically by the epileptologist while closely monitoring the patient for seizure reoccurrence.

As with RNS, DBS implantation requires a two-part cranial surgery. During the first part of the surgery, two EEG depth leads are placed deep inside the brain through small holes made in the skull. Using image guidance and computerized stereotactic technology and MRI or computed tomography (CT), the neurosurgeon will map the brain to implant the electrodes in the correct positions (Fig. 24, pg. 100). Since each person's brain is different, mapping can take anywhere from 30 minutes to 2 hours for each side of the brain. Once the correct target sites are confirmed, the permanent DBS electrodes will be inserted and tested for about 20 minutes. The testing process focuses on any unwanted stimulation-induced side effects, which, unlike the beneficial effects of DBS, will be present immediately. During this time, the neurosurgeon will purposefully turn up the stimulation to a higher intensity than normally used in order to deliberately produce any adverse stimulation-induced side effects. These include tingling in the arm or leg, difficulty speaking, a pulling sensation in the tongue or face, or flashing lights. The sensations felt during the testing process can be mildly uncomfortable for the patient but not painful. The electrodes will be then connected to wires that are tunneled under the skin, behind the ear, and inside the skin of the neck down to the chest, where they are attached to the neurostimulator (Fig. 25, pg. 102). The neurosurgeon or surgical nurse will then program the stimulator using a hand-held computer to set the frequency and intensity of electrical stimulation delivered.

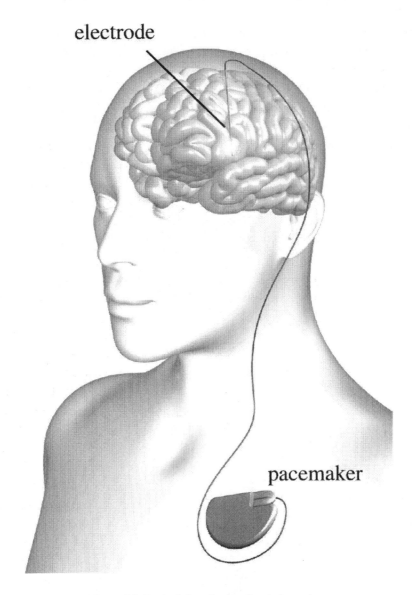

Figure 24: Typical deep brain stimulation setup.
(Shamir R, Noecker A and McIntyre C [CC BY 3.0]/Wikimedia Commons)

As with RNS and other cranial procedures, risks with DBS include a 1–2 percent chance of stroke due to bleeding and a 5 percent chance of infection, neurological impairment, and, most commonly, self-limiting headache and mild pain at the implant site. Some patients also report paresthesia (feeling "pins and needles"), memory problems, and depression after DBS surgery. These side effects are usually temporary and diminish over time. Similar to VNS and RNS, patients with DBS implants must avoid MRI scans to avoid causing damage to the neurostimulator.

In the weeks that follow DBS surgery, the patient's progress will be carefully monitored in order to make necessary adjustments to the stimulation. It can take months to find the right level of electrical stimulation because it will vary for every person. The patient will also receive a magnet that he or she can use to turn the stimulation on or off by holding it up to the neurostimulator. Battery life for the DBS system is about 3–4 years, depending on frequency and intensity of stimulation delivered.

Current research indicates that electrical stimulation therapies like VNS, RNS, and DBS offer a more promising future for patients with medically refractory epilepsy for whom resective surgery is not a viable option.

Newer targets for electrical stimulation are now being tested, such as trigeminal nerve stimulation or stimulation of other brain structures, and new noninvasive methods are being tested such as skin stimulation. Although complete seizure control is uncommon, electrical stimulation treatments in carefully selected cases can offer improved quality of life for these patients by reducing seizure frequency and intensity and providing a chance of lowering medication. For the patient considering electrical stimulation therapy, the decision to undergo invasive surgery is one that should be made after careful consideration of the possible risks, benefits, and other concerns he or she may have. Patients should also consider the risks of not doing the surgery and the danger of continued, uncontrolled epilepsy. The patient and family should have an in-depth conversation with his or her epileptologist and neurosurgeon, nurse practitioner, and any other members of the medical team available to speak in order to prepare mentally and emotionally for the surgical process. Tips, including an outline of frequently asked questions on how to make an educated and sound decision for surgery are discussed in the following chapter.

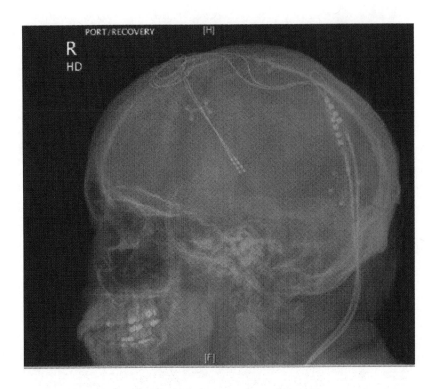

Figure 25: Skull x-ray of DBS implant. The leads shown in the x-ray are implanted in both thalami and connected by cables to a stimulator in the chest wall.
(Dr. Robert Fisher/Stanford University)

CHAPTER SIX
COMING TO A DECISION ON SURGERY

- The surgical consultation is the patient's opportunity to understand the procedure, ask questions, and get to know the neurosurgeon and his or her medical team.
- Weighing surgery risks against potential benefits is a very important step when making a decision to have epilepsy surgery.
- Understanding the implications of a life without surgery and risks associated with uncontrolled seizures is also important to weigh in the decision.
- Preparing emotionally and mentally to have surgery, go through recovery, and live with the results is equally as important to make a sound choice.

The Process

Once all the necessary pre-surgical testing is completed, a patient's case is presented at a multidisciplinary conference (MDC) before a final decision is made. Here, a group of neurologists, neurosurgeons, neuropsychologists, psychiatrists, and sometimes imaging specialists discuss each patient's individual case to reach a decision regarding whether surgery is a good idea or not, and, if yes, what type of surgery, if any, is most likely to provide seizure freedom. If the panel concludes that the patient is a viable candidate for surgery, it will next be up to the patient to decide what choice is personally best. The decision to have surgery requires a patient to carefully consider a number of factors, from both a medical and personal standpoint. Weighing the potential benefits and risks associated with surgery against a life plagued with uncontrolled seizures is pertinent to making a sound decision about what is best for you. It is vital that a patient fully understands the potential outcome for his or her personal situation by talking to his or her medical team, family, and other care providers. This chapter will outline the important points to consider, potential questions you may have, and how to decide whether surgery is right for you.

Surgical Consultation
The first step in reaching a decision to have epilepsy surgery is meeting with the neurosurgeon during the surgical consultation. At this point, the patient will have already met with his or her epileptologist to discuss the decision reached at the MDC, and he or she will know which type of surgery is likely

to offer the best outcome for seizure control. The neurosurgeon will further discuss the specifics of the surgery and explain in detail the potential benefits and risks associated with it. This meeting is also a crucial time for the patient and his or her family to become acquainted with the operating surgeon and ask any questions they may have, both to feel at ease with the procedure as well as to become fully comfortable with the head physician leading the operating team through the surgery. The surgical consultation is an integral opportunity for the patient to gather as much information as possible to feel fully equipped to make a sound decision regarding surgery. It is also a time for the surgeon to help quell any anxieties, worries, and concerns the patient and his or her family may have about surgery, and patients are always recommended to bring a list of any questions or concerns they may have to this visit. Common topics you can expect to discuss during the surgical consultation are outlined next.

The Procedure

Certainly, one of the most important things the patient will need to understand on a basic level is the general steps of the procedure to take place. Without going into too many details, the surgeon will walk you through what will happen during the operation, what will be removed or implanted, and about how long the entire procedure will last. A brain surgery is involved with resective surgery, RNS, and DBS, all of which require the patient to be put asleep with general anesthesia, which also factors into the length of the full procedure. It is best not to get overwhelmed with the minute details of the procedure because they may likely be too complex to comprehend fully. The important takeaway from this portion of the consultation is that the patient largely understands the general scope of the surgery and what it hopes to accomplish and why so that he or she feels as prepared as possible.

Understanding Surgical Benefits and Risks

An equally important part of the surgical consultation is for the patient to know what benefits he or she can possibly anticipate from surgery compared to the potential risks. As discussed in Chapter 4 and Chapter 5, possible benefits and risks vary with each surgery, with resective surgery yielding the highest chances of becoming completely seizure-free. With that said, each patient's case is unique, and certain people may be at a higher risk for complications depending on age, any other pre-existing health conditions, allergies, or complications from previous surgeries. For that reason, a patient may consider the risks of surgery to outweigh the potential benefits of becoming seizure-free or having fewer seizures.

On the other hand, a patient whose quality of life is very poor due to the debilitating consequences of having uncontrolled seizures may feel that the potential benefits of epilepsy surgery greatly outweigh the risks. There is no true right answer, as the decision to have surgery is as much emotional as it is rational, and it belongs to each patient. With that said, however, the neurosurgeon can provide great insight into what is the likely outcome from surgery versus the potential outcome to help the patient make a more informed decision.

Something else very important to consider is the level of expertise and years of experience your neurosurgeon has in performing the specific type of surgery you may be having. Don't be afraid to ask any questions you may have regarding your surgeon's experience with similar cases and how he or she may handle complications if any arise. At least when it comes to resective surgery, most surgeons generally lean toward being conservative when removing tissue.

Even so, it is a patient's prerogative to know first-stand where his or her surgeon stands when dealing with surgical complications. Feeling completely comfortable with your medical team cannot be understated, and it is ultimately up to the patient to gather as much information as he or she needs to fully trust the neurosurgeon and his team. There may be an option to speak with the surgeon's previous patients about their own surgery experiences, and it is highly recommended that patients take advantage of this resource if available.

Understanding Recovery and Life After Surgery

One of the biggest fears patients have about epilepsy surgery is what they will experience during recovery and how long it will take to heal completely. As discussed in the previous chapter, each epilepsy surgery involves a different procedure and varies in the amount of invasiveness; subsequently, recovery for every individual surgery also varies, with resective surgery typically involving the longest and most intense recovery process. In addition to understanding the actual surgical procedure, the surgical consultation will allow for the neurosurgeon to explain the subsequent recovery in detail. It is important to remember that even though the surgeon can offer a general explanation of the recovery period, any unforeseen surgery complications can affect how quickly the patient will fully heal. Understanding this should not be a reason to feel more alarmed or nervous, but rather it is a way for the patient to know what he or she can expect in the days and weeks following surgery. This is another reason why speaking to previous patients can be very beneficial to help calm any nerves, because previous patients can offer an invaluable first-person perspective that even a highly experienced neurosurgeon can not.

Additionally, the neurosurgeon will have a team of specialized surgery care providers with whom you will have the opportunity to meet and talk before the surgery. This team, usually made up of licensed nurses and/or nurse practitioners, will be available to address recovery questions or concerns during and after the surgery. It is also this team that will most likely help explain the specifics of what recovery will entail, including the pain, discomfort, and any other common issues.

Patients will see the neurosurgeon immediately following surgery, during the hospital stay, and for a follow-up visit in the few weeks after. However, the surgeon's team of nurses and nurse practitioners will most likely be the point persons for the patient's recovery care, and they will be able to offer valuable information to both the patient and his or her family regarding recovery.

Patients should take the opportunity to speak to every person who will be in charge of their post-surgical care to further educate themselves on surgery before making a decision. The more knowledge you have, the more certain you will be that you are making the best decision for you.

Life Without Surgery

When making the decision whether to have surgery, patients with medically refractory epilepsy who are viable candidates for surgery should fully understand the implications of choosing not to have surgery. As mentioned previously in earlier chapters, resective surgery is the most comprehensive solution available today to correct a seizure disorder. It is also not considered the "last resort" solution to epilepsy it once was; instead, surgery is an option to deal with uncontrolled seizures effectively and to address a number of issues and risks that patients commonly deal with every day. In the following sections, we address some of the most common issues and risk of persistent seizures.

Cognitive Damage

For patients for whom antiepileptic drugs (AEDs) have failed, the subsequent cognitive damage from uncontrolled seizures can range from short-term memory loss to the inability to find words while speaking or the difficulty performing tasks involving executive function. Depending on where the seizures originate and if they spread, various parts of the brain and their related functions can suffer. For younger people especially, this is an important consequence to keep in mind when making the decision to have surgery. Continuous damage to such vital brain functions can be very detrimental to patients still in school or in the early state of their careers, when learning new skills and retaining new information constantly are the norms. However, dealing with cognitive damage can be extremely difficult for anyone suffering from uncontrolled seizures. Everyday functions like remembering names or finding the right words during conversation can take a toll because of seizure damage, and these functions can continue to weaken over time if seizures are left uncontrolled. Mood disorders such as depression and dysthymia have also been linked to epilepsy, and their implications, too, can greatly impact a person's day-to-day activities very negatively.

Medication Side Effects

Many patients with medically refractory epilepsy deal with an additional burden of being heavily medicated with AEDs, which can often cause side effects that compound the difficulties of having uncontrolled seizures. Some common AED side effects like drowsiness, headache, and nausea can even make day-to-day life more difficult, which is an important factor to weigh when considering surgery. Of course, side effects will vary from patient to patient and from medication to medication. For epilepsy patients whose daily life is both a struggle against uncontrolled seizures and medication side effects, opting for surgery might be an easier decision. However, it is also important to discuss with your doctor if your AED regimen poses any long-term risk to your health, or, for women planning to get pregnant, whether it is safe to do so while taking AEDs. Often, the doses of medication can impact the extent of side effects a patient experiences or any other risks he or she may face, but it is also common with patients with medically refractory epilepsy generally to be on higher doses of AEDs to help control their seizures. For such reasons, it is worth weighing how much, if at all, of a negative impact AEDs are having on other areas of your life when making the decision for epilepsy surgery. Especially for prospective surgery candidates, a successful operation could mean a significant reduction in medication intake, if not a complete end to taking medications daily.

Disability and Lower Quality of Life

Perhaps one of the biggest factors patients must weigh when considering epilepsy surgery is how debilitating the condition is for them. Life with uncontrolled seizures can mean a life with numerous disabilities, some not so obvious as others. For example, adult patients who live with frequent and unpredictable seizures must rely on public transportation and/or their families and friends to get around. Most states even have laws set in place that restrict people from obtaining a driver's license or maintaining their driver's license if they are known to have seizures regularly. This can be a very difficult situation for both the patient and his or her support network. Without the ability to drive or operate any motor vehicle, adult patients often feel a great sense of dependence on others, creating a situation that is both financially taxing and emotionally straining. For younger patients with epilepsy, never having the opportunity to learn to drive or travel alone can also be very difficult and can sometimes hinder their natural maturation into adulthood.

Additionally, epilepsy patients must consider the other risks they face on a day-to-day basis and how much of an impact they have on reducing their quality of life. Injury is usually the primary concern, and sometimes there is very little that can be done to prevent it. Falling, picking up sharp objects, and walking into harm's way are all very real dangers epilepsy patients face while dealing with uncontrolled seizures. While there are some precautions you can take to prevent harm, such as safeguarding the area around your work desk or avoiding the use of sharp utensils during meals, it is nearly impossible to anticipate every danger. Living life with such a debilitating disability can take a physical, mental, and emotional toll on the patient, and it is important that he or she consider just how much of an impact this has on his or her quality of life when considering surgery.

Sudden Unexpected Death

The most serious risk to consider when making the decision to have epilepsy surgery is the possibility of *sudden unexpected death in epilepsy,* or SUDEP. This cause of death is categorized as such because the person can otherwise be called healthy, and no other cause of death can be found during the autopsy.

More than 1 in 2,000 epilepsy patients die from SUDEP each year. The risk is greater for people who suffer from uncontrolled seizures, increasing to 1 in 150 patients. SUDEP is rare in children but remains the leading cause of death in young adults with certain types of uncontrolled epilepsy. Patients who suffer from severe generalized epilepsies are also known to have increased risk for SUDEP.

Because doctors know very little about what causes SUDEP, there is also little that can be done to prevent it, other than to prevent the seizures. The death often occurs during sleep, and there is not always evidence that a seizure has occurred.

Getting Ready for Surgery:
Mental and Emotional Readiness

One final consideration during the decision-making process is whether you are mentally and emotionally prepared for the surgery, the recovery, and the days following. Even if the patient has weighed his or her options thoroughly with the help of his or her family and medical team, it is ultimately a personal decision that no one else can make. There may be a clear answer on paper, but it is equally as important that the patient feel mentally and emotionally ready to endure through the stresses of what surgery can entail. The burden of making a decision in itself can be stressful, so it is advisable for the patient to do as much homework as needed to prepare emotionally. Recognizing the common stressors ahead of time can be helpful.

Not wanting to be disappointed yet again, for example, patients sometimes struggle with where to set their expectations going into surgery, especially after a prolonged struggle to find a solution for uncontrolled seizures. Worries about being put to sleep with anesthesia or nervousness about surgery in general can also get in the way of making a sound decision, but they are all normal feelings to have prior to any procedure. The best a patient can do to alleviate these worries is to thoroughly exhaust his or her options for information gathering. Talking to the medical team is vital to feel at ease with the doctors and nurses who will be operating on you and taking care of you during and after the surgery, but it is equally advisable to seek out other types of support to calm nerves. Speaking openly about surgery with family and friends is very helpful for some patients, as is speaking to a therapist or counselor. Because many patients do have some fear of death in surgery, they may reach out to an authority figure in their church or spiritual community to help quell these fears. Even still, some people find the greatest comfort in speaking with former patients who have gone through the entire process and who are happy to fill in the information gaps that no one else may be able to do other than someone who has gone through epilepsy surgery first-hand. Whatever the fear or worry, it is pertinent to keep in mind that it is perfectly normal to have some anxiety before any surgery, much less one that involves the brain. What is more important is whether the patient can also feel comfortable and confident in the decision to proceed with surgery and recovery, more of which will be discussed in detail in the next chapter.

CHAPTER SEVEN
PREPARING FOR AND RECOVERING FROM RESECTIVE SURGERY

- Certain medical and personal preparations should begin in the week(s) leading up to surgery.
- Establishing the roles family and friends ahead of time is key to preparation and to ease anxiety about surgery and recovery.
- The day of surgery will begin very early for you. Family and friends should prepare for a normal course of events for the day.
- Recovery will span 4–8 weeks, from the time in the hospital to recovering at home. Expectations and tips are discussed.
- Follow-up visits will continue over the weeks/months following surgery before any decisions are made to reduce seizure medication.

Once a patient has come to the decision that surgery is the next best step in his or her seizure treatment, it's important to prepare for what to expect in the days leading up to surgery and the recovery period. Resective surgery recovery, in particular, can be a very strenuous process, with many steps along the way. This chapter will discuss how best to prepare for surgery, normal expectations for recovery, and important tips on how to make the process easier.

Week(s) Before Surgery

In the last days before surgery, daily life can become somewhat hectic. There will be many arrangements to make, from finalizing insurance approval to taking leave from work or school. Asking for help from a family or friend is advised because the preparations can compound any stress that you may already be feeling about the pending operation. The next sections detail some preparations you can expect to make in the final days before surgery.

Medical Preparations
In the weeks leading up to surgery, there will be very few changes made to a patient's seizure treatment regimen. In particular, you should continue to take anti-epileptic drugs (AEDs) as prescribed by your specialist and monitor seizure activity as normal. The key change in daily routine will be to stop taking aspirin, any anti-inflammatory drugs, and herbal medications at least 2 weeks prior to the scheduled operation. If a patient is taking

aspirin or is prescribed an anti-inflammatory drug for another condition, it will be extremely important to relay this information to the neurosurgeon and his medical team during pre-surgical consultation. In general, aspirin and similar medications and certain over-the-counter (OTC) vitamins and supplements may need to be discontinued a week to 10 days before surgery. For example, fish supplements may increase bleeding and should be discontinued a week before surgery.

Additionally, patients are advised to speak to their primary care physician and/or other specialists to discuss a medication regimen going into surgery. Certain drugs may have the potential of creating complications during a major operation, and it's important that you are completely honest about any medications, vitamins, or supplements that you are taking to help the medical team properly address them before the surgery.

Personal Preparations

Perhaps more important in the weeks leading up to surgery will be the various preparations a patient will need to make concerning his or her personal life. It will be extremely helpful to create a checklist for yourself to identify certain arrangements to make while you are away for surgery and recovery, as well as any other loose ends to tie up. It is pertinent that you avoid stress in order to recover properly, so it is that much more important to take care of as many odds and ends before surgery. Some questions to address on the checklist can include:

- *Are my supervisors at work/school aware of the surgery date and how much time I'm expected to be away?*

- *Is there a designated person who is in charge of communicating any changes to my expected return date to work/school should there be any?*

- *Is there a designated person who is in charge of keeping nonimmediate family and friends updated with news during and following the surgery?*

- *Are there any miscellaneous arrangements I need to make beforehand, such as paying bills or rent?*

- *Have all the financial arrangements been made for medical bills, and has my insurance company cleared the surgery?*

- *Do visiting family and friends know when and where they can come to visit during the hospital stay?*

- *Is there anyone else I see in my daily life (i.e., roommates, neighbors, coworkers, friends) I should tell about my surgery, so they don't worry when I'm gone and/or return from the hospital?*

- *Am I experiencing any last-minute anxiety about surgery that should be addressed with the medical team, a therapist, or family and friends?*

- *Have I taken care of any legal issues including power of attorney, financial arrangements, and a living will?*

Remember, the key takeaway from these questions is to anticipate situations in which you may need be present and make arrangements to address them to avoid any unnecessary stress later. It will be pertinent that you are in a relaxed environment following surgery, so whatever can be taken care of beforehand should be done so.

The Night Before Surgery

As the day of surgery approaches, you will have a few more last-minute preparations to make before the procedure. A major operation like a craniotomy will almost always start very early in the morning, so it is best to be fully ready to go to the hospital the night before. The preparations to make are similar in nature to those made in the weeks leading up to surgery and are discussed here.

Medical Preparations
Patients should continue to take AEDs as prescribed the night before surgery. It is also fine to eat and drink as normal, but a lighter meal is better the night before surgery. The one very important rule to follow in preparation for surgery is to avoid eating or drinking anything (including water) after midnight of the night before the procedure. Patients undergoing resective surgery will also be given antimicrobial shampoo or wipes by the surgical team to help prepare the surgical site the night before. This product should be applied as instructed during the surgical consultation.

Personal Preparations
By the night before surgery, you should have very few preparations still left to make. At this point, it should be a matter of double-checking that all your arrangements are in order for the next morning and getting some rest. Because the procedure will be scheduled very early, and you and your family will need to be at the hospital for pre-admission tests a couple of hours before that, it is not uncommon to get very little sleep. Some last-minute nerves will also likely set in the night before, and it's important to remember that this is a very normal occurrence.

Many people naturally have a fear of the hospital or feel nervous undergoing any medical procedure, let alone a very invasive one like epilepsy surgery. Reminding yourself that some level of anxiety and nervousness is extremely common, even for patients for whom surgery was an "easy" decision, is helpful for maintaining a positive attitude. This is also an important time to allow family and friends to help keep you from focusing too much on the surgery, and it's highly recommended that you do something fun and relaxing the night before the procedure. When it's time to get final preparations in order, you can refer to the following checklist of questions.

- *Does my hospital bag have my toiletries, warm pajamas and/or bathrobe, glasses and/or contact lenses with case, and medication for the morning?*
  - o <u>Remember:</u> Do not take anything of value or large sums of money with you to the hospital. Laptops, tablets, and cell phones are allowed, and you should bring them along with any necessary power chargers if they will help make your hospital stay more comfortable. Reading material is also highly recommended.
- *Have I designated someone in charge of relaying information to other family and friends?*
  - o This person should be a close family member or friend who will be directly in touch with the surgical team at the hospital on the day of surgery. It is best that you ask one or two people to be in charge of communicating to other family and friends any updates throughout the day so as to avoid any unnecessary worry.
- *Do I know how I'm getting to the hospital?*
  - o Most likely you will be traveling with a close family member or friend on the morning of your surgery. It's a good idea to know exactly who that will be and how you will be traveling to the hospital. You will be notified by the hospital's admissions office when and where to report in the morning. For patients who are riding with a driver, it's advised that you ask about parking arrangements well ahead of time because they will differ with every hospital. Plan for delays, and leave early to make sure you arrive for pre-admission testing on time.

The Morning of Surgery and Procedure

Often, the day of surgery can be a whirlwind of emotions for patients and those close to them. By this point, you have been through weeks or possibly months of pre-surgical exams, consultations, and preparations. For some, the morning of surgery can be very exciting, especially considering the possibility of being seizure-free in the near future. It is important to remember that a positive attitude and continued support from family and friends in the final hours before surgery can make a big difference in settling anxiety for everyone. With that said, it is of equal importance that you be able to maintain realistic expectations for not only long-term results, but also especially for what is to come in the immediate days following surgery. Attentive care—both medical and emotional—will be vital during this time for a proper recovery. Here, we discuss a normal course of events on the day of surgery and realistic expectations for the patient and those close to him or her.

Pre-admission Testing

Once you arrive at the hospital for the pre-admission testing, you will be taken through a series of routine tests before meeting with the anesthesiologist and neurosurgeon to go over the surgical plan once more and to ask any last questions. You will be asked to sign a consent form for surgery and anesthesia after this meeting. A few family or friends are allowed to accompany you during the pre-admission testing and wait together in the surgical holding area. The designated contact person for the surgical team should be present at this time to ask any last-minute questions and simply for general knowledge of what is happening before the surgery. You can expect the following tests and events during this time, but in some centers, if the pre-admission tests marked with asterisks have been completed within a week of the surgery date, they will not be repeated:

- Change into hospital gown
- Wash hair with antimicrobial shampoo
- Routine blood work: CBC (blood count), PT/PTT (clotting factors), SMAG (liver function, chemistry)
- Urinalysis*
- Electrocardiogram (EKG)
- History and physical exam
- Interview with the anesthesiologist (to discuss generally what will happen during surgery)
- Possible chest X-ray
- Meeting with the neurosurgeon

Once testing is completed, you will have one more opportunity to speak to your family and friends before being taken to the operating room. Your belongings must be given to the waiting family and friends because the surgical team is not responsible for them. There will be an opportunity later to place them in your recovery room, as instructed by hospital staff. At this point, you will receive any further instructions in the operating room from the surgical team. Most likely, you will immediately see the anesthesiologist whom you met with during the pre-admission period, who will guide you through further steps. You may also see your neurosurgeon and other members of the surgical team. Once the general anesthesia has been administered, you will quickly fall asleep. Usually this is the last memory you will have before surgery, and all other prepping will continue after you are asleep (Fig. 26, pg. 118).

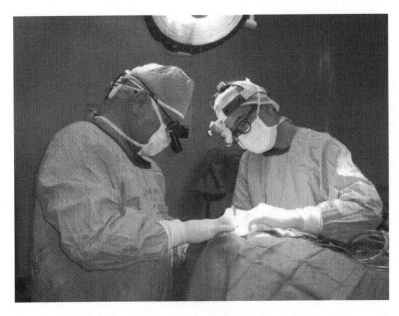

Figure 26: Neurosurgeons operating on patient in the OR.
(Dr. Ruben Kuzniecky/NYU)

Expectations for Family and Friends
During the Procedure

Once the surgical team has taken you into the operating room, a member of the surgical team will direct family and friends to a designated waiting area. The neurosurgeon will have already spoken with the family and/or friends who accompanied the patient to the hospital for surgery, and he or she will instruct them where to wait for news. A nurse or nurse liaison will come here to give updates during the surgery, but waiting family and friends are also encouraged to walk around, eat, and occupy themselves otherwise while waiting. The surgeon will most likely call them personally if they are not in the waiting area once surgery is over, so there is no need to worry about missing an update.

The role of family and friends should not go unappreciated during this time, especially because it can sometimes be just as stressful if not more so to be the ones waiting to hear any surgery updates. It's especially important to remember that surgery time can fall into a range (about 5–8 hours), and a longer-than-expected surgery does not necessarily indicate complications. Any number of factors can cause a delay in surgery, and it's best to assume that everything is okay until otherwise notified. Something else to keep in mind is whether the patient is having single-stage or multistage surgery, because the latter requires much more time. Generally, family and friends can anticipate periodic updates:

1. Start of Surgery:
Once surgery has officially begun, a nurse or nurse liaison will let waiting family and friends know that the procedure has started. This is often a good time to get something to eat and find a comfortable place to wait because it may be a while before the next update.

2. Midpoint:
Sometimes the surgeon will take a short break about halfway through the surgery, and he or she may offer an update personally. Otherwise, waiting family and friends can expect to hear from the nurse or nurse liaison.

3. End of Surgery:
Once the surgery is over, the neurosurgeon will speak to the patient's

waiting family and friends personally and offer further instructions on when and where they can see the patient. If the patient is having a multistage surgery, a timeline for the next procedure will be given.

4. Immediately Following Surgery:

The events immediately following surgery will likely be a blur for you because you will have been under anesthesia for quite some time. The following paragraphs outline the general timeline of post-surgery, but you should be aware that you will likely not remember the hours immediately after surgery. Having an idea of what to expect during this time is beneficial simply for your general knowledge.

Waking up in the Operating Room and Post-Anesthesia Care Unit (PACU) Recovery

Once the procedure is completely finished, you will be awakened in the operating room by the anesthesiologist. The breathing tube used during surgery will be removed, although you may have an oxygen mask or nasal prongs in the nose briefly until you are more awake. Several IVs will also remain to provide fluids, as well as an arterial line in the wrist to monitor blood pressure continuously. A Foley catheter will stay in place for at least another day to drain urine. In addition to the EKG, you will be connected to a portable electroencephalogram (EEG) immediately following surgery so any seizures can be recorded.

At this point, you will be moved to the post-anesthesia care unit (PACU), where you will stay until more awake and able to talk and follow simple commands. The waiting family and/or friends will be allowed to see you briefly during this time, but it's likely that you will have little to no memory of the visit, even if you are somewhat responsive. You can also expect to see the neurosurgeon at some point during this period. In addition to waking up from the anesthesia, you will be given pain medications that have a sedative effect. The combination of both will make you very sleepy, and it will be normal to be a little incoherent at this time. A specially trained PACU nurse will closely monitor you vital signs and fluid balance every 15 minutes. A PACU nurse practitioner will also perform frequent neurological checks, while an anesthesiologist will continue to monitor you as the anesthesia wears off. Once you are deemed recovered from the anesthesia, you will be discharged to the neurosurgery intensive care unit (NSICU).

Neurosurgery ICU Recovery

Patients will spend one or two nights after surgery in the NSICU. Unless there were complications during the surgery, you will be moved to a regular room on the neurosurgery ward the next day. Visits are allowed, but they should be kept to a minimum. One family member may stay overnight if needed. It is necessary for you to rest and sleep the first night after surgery because it can be one of the most physically uncomfortable stages of recovery. A specially trained nurse will be there to administer pain medications and ease the discomfort as best as possible. The best you can do to prepare is to remember that your brain is recovering from a very invasive surgery, and it will take some time for it to heal. That process can be difficult, but knowing what to expect can help immensely. The NSICU recovery may include.

Extreme Nausea:

Nausea is one of the most common side effects of the pain medications you will receive. Headaches may still persist, and, combined with the fact that you will not have eaten in nearly 24 hours, it is extremely likely that you will experience intense nausea in the NSIC. Anti-nausea medication can be given in this case to help. You will be advised to try to avoid vomiting because it causes pressure to the head. Even with the anti-nausea medication, however, you may feel very sick and vomit. This is very common, and you are encouraged to communicate the level of pain and discomfort in order to receive the right medications in a timely manner. It's important to ask for medication at the onset of discomfort because it will take longer for the drugs to work once the pain becomes worse.

Strong Headaches:

Even with pain medications, you may experience headaches throughout the night as the medications wear off. You will receive steroids to help decrease inflammation and brain swelling, and the dose will decrease slowly over the next week, until it is tapered off completely after leaving the hospital. Depending on how you are tolerating the side effects of one pain medication, the nurse may try another. It's also important to remember that IV drugs will take effect more quickly but cannot be given as frequently. For this reason, the nurse may offer you pain pills and/or an ice pack to help ease pain in between the IV drugs.

General Discomfort:

Although you will be advised to rest and sleep for the first night, it can be very difficult to do so. You will be awakened periodically by a nurse to check vitals and perform other routine monitoring, which, in combination with the pain, can make it difficult to sleep. Again, it's helpful to remember that this is all a normal part of recovery (Fig. 27, pg. 124).

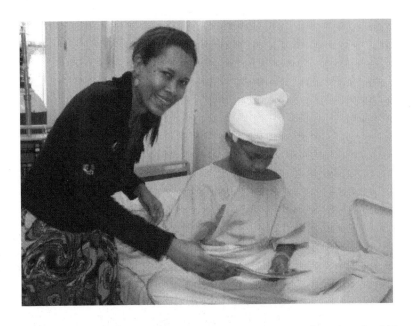

Figure 27: Though patients may experience pain and discomfort, they should be
able to engage in some activities like sitting up and reading,
as soon as the first day of surgery.
(Dr. Ruben Kuzniecky, NYU)

Hospital Recovery After NSICU

One day after surgery, you will be taken for a magnetic resonance imaging (MRI) session in some centers. The loud noises in the machine can cause intense discomfort, and it's best if you communicate this to the nurse. In most cases, you will be moved to a regular hospital room the morning after the NSICU and spend the next 1–3 days here before being discharged. The neurosurgery nurse practitioner will visit daily to monitor progress, answer questions, and manage your care with the multidisciplinary team of doctors, nurses, and therapists. The neurosurgeon and other doctors will also come by every day or every other day. During this time, you will continue to experience intermittent headaches, but the pain and nausea in particular should begin to subside considerably. Normal occurrences and tips for this period of recovery include:

Mobility and Motor Functions:
You will feel general weakness following surgery, but moving around in bed will be encouraged. Bedside physical and occupational therapy will begin the first day after surgery, and you will be given exercises to do in bed to promote deep breathing and circulation. Compression socks will also be worn to promote blood circulation in the legs. When you feel strong enough, you will be encouraged to take walks around the room or hospital floor with assistance. For the most part, you will have good control over motor functions and be able to move around freely (Fig. 28, pg. 127).

Hygiene:
Showering with assistance will be an option after moving to the regular hospital floor, but you will need to be careful to keep the head area dry for at least 5 days. Keeping up other daily hygiene routines like brushing your teeth and washing your face is recommended because these can greatly help you start to regain a sense of normalcy in an otherwise stressful situation.

Eating and Drinking:
You are encouraged to begin eating light, bland foods at this point. It's likely that you will not have eaten anything for more than 24 hours. Although it may take a few days to regain an appetite, eating foods like fruit, crackers, and oatmeal is a good place to start. Drinking on your own will have begun right after surgery, and you should continue to have fluids to stay hydrated. Juice, smoothies, and milk are also good recommendations to provide nutrition, especially if your appetite hasn't returned.

Energy:
You should expect to feel fatigued after surgery, especially in the first week.

With that said, light exercise is highly suggested not only to regain strength and promote healthy physiological functions but also to refresh your mind.

Digestion:
As previously mentioned, it can take a few days to regain an appetite after brain surgery. In combination with the medications and lack of exercise and good nutrition, you may begin to feel very lethargic. Poor digestion and constipation can be a result of all these factors. If needed, nurses can offer fiber supplements and/or laxatives to promote bowel movements.

Noise Sensitivity:
Often after a craniotomy, a patient may experience noise sensitivity in the ear on the side where he or she was operated. This will likely get better over time but can sometimes make you prone to more headaches while recovering.

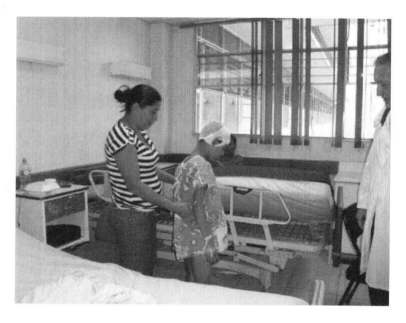

Figure 28: Doctor testing patient's motor functions in the days following surgery.
(Dr. Ruben Kuzniecky/NYU)

Hospital Discharge and At-Home Care

After about 1–3 days in the hospital following the final procedure, you will be discharged to continue recovering at home. There can sometimes be some anxiety associated with leaving the hospital because you will not feel fully recovered. Although it will likely take at least a few more weeks for you to begin to feel "normal" again, there is no reason to worry about going home. You will only be discharged when you are deemed no longer in need of daily medical care, although both physical and emotional support from close family and/or friends will be vital in the weeks and months to come. Expectations and advice for at-home recovery include:

Daily Activities:
As in the hospital, you will be highly encouraged to resume normal day-to-day activities as best as you can without overdoing it. Proper healing requires a balance of rest and light exercise, so it is very important to establish a routine of incorporating both. You should be extra careful to avoid any heavy lifting, straining, or applying pressure to the head. Frequent periods of rest and naps are recommended, as is getting at least 8 hours of sleep every night. It will likely take anywhere from 2 to 4 weeks for fatigue to completely resolve. Most patients are not ready to return to work or school for at least 4–6 weeks, though depending on the type of job, it's possible to resume work remotely or part-time a few weeks after surgery. You should consult the surgeon and epileptologist first to make sure that you are ready to resume work/school. Whatever the case, it is critical that you take the proper time to fully recover and avoid unnecessary physical and mental stress. Additionally, a healthy diet of nutritious foods will help considerably in regaining strength and energy.

Pain Management:
Mild to moderate headaches should be expected for at least a couple more weeks after returning home. You may especially experience more pain in the first few days after being discharged as the steroids are tapered off completely. You should have prescription pain medication from the doctor that can be taken for the pain. (Acetaminophen or ibuprofen is a suggested alternative if the pain isn't very strong.) Some patients report less energy and sometimes feeling sad during this time. Other side effects reported include increased appetite and difficulty falling asleep, all of which should

go away within 2–3 days after steroids are stopped. Whether to take prescription pain medication or OTC medication depends on each patient, and he or she should take what personally feels necessary.

Wound Care:

The surgical wound does not need any particular care until the staples are taken out by the neurosurgeon. Until then, only baby shampoo should be used daily to keep the wound clean. Nothing should be put on the suture line, including any other types of hair products. If necessary, a gauze pad can be placed on the wound with a stockinette. You should make sure to carefully observe the wound for signs of infection such as redness, swelling, drainage, and worsening discomfort.

Mood:

Attention to mental and emotional wellness should not be overlooked in the process of recovery. Rather, ensuring that you maintain a positive attitude throughout surgery and recovery will be instrumental for faster and better healing. With that said, it is equally important to understand that a healing brain can create a roller coaster of emotions for you. In combination with all of the aforementioned factors that make recovery already stressful, it is normal for patients to feel a sense of sadness and even hopelessness at times. Caretakers should be sensitive to this and contact the neurosurgery team if the patient becomes increasingly depressed. For the patient, simply being prepared for this phase of recovery can greatly help you be self-aware of the "tricks" your brain can play, thereby allowing for better control of your emotions. Additionally, reminding yourself that it is your brain healing that is causing you to feel this way can help to separate yourself from the emotions and address them more productively.

"Foggy" Head:

Perhaps the greatest factor of a craniotomy recovery that can exaggerate all other symptoms is the feeling of a "foggy" or "cloudy" head. Though all patients may have their own unique way of explaining this sometimes-indescribable feeling, one common denominator is the feeling of "fogginess" in the head. Another way to imagine it is the "heavy head" feeling that accompanies the flu without the other flu symptoms. What is especially important to note about this symptom is that it can exaggerate the feeling of fatigue and sadness that you may already be experiencing. Additionally, it can be the one symptom of recovery that outlasts pain, taking between 4–8 weeks to go away completely. While it may not seem very intimidating, the feeling of "foggy" head can make you feel like you are constantly in a state of illness, which in turn can cause frustration and sadness. Prescription pain medications can contribute to this feeling, though you should remember that the fogginess more directly stems from the brain healing itself. It will go away in due time, and patience can go a long way during this period.

Post-surgical Follow-Ups:
There may be multiple follow-ups for the next 6 months to several years to monitor progress. Patients can expect the basic timeline of events following surgery:

Removing Stitches/Staples:
You will visit with the neurosurgery team 7–10 days after the surgery for a postoperative check-up and to have the stitches/staples in the surgical wound removed. The timeline may be longer or shorter depending on your case and the surgeon's preference. For a multistage operation, the surgeon will likely remove stitches/staples after 2 weeks. Depending on what has been used to close up the wound, you may experience little to moderate pain during this process. Pain medication and/or nausea medication may be offered.

Changes in Seizure Medication:
There will be no changes made to your seizure medication regimen immediately following surgery. You will continue to take medication as normal through recovery. Changes to the medication dose, if any, will be made only after a follow-up EEG shows no epileptic activity and your epileptologist deems it appropriate. This will not happen for at least several months (3–6 months). In the meantime, it is extremely important for both you and your family/friends to monitor any seizure activity and report it immediately to the team. Over the long term, most patients who stay seizure-free will reduce seizure medications, but the timing, doses, and the like are completely individualized to the patient's condition.

EEG Follow-Up:

The epileptologist may order a routine or ambulatory EEG about 2 weeks to 3 months after hospital discharge to get a better idea of epileptic activity and to compare to the EEG done before surgery. Sometimes, patients are unable to know for sure whether they are having seizures (especially those who have partial seizures), so the EEG's results can provide a clearer picture of any abnormal activity. It is very important to note that because the brain is still very much healing this soon after surgery, an inconclusive EEG may not necessarily mean you are having seizures. Its purpose is more to provide an understanding of how the brain waves are behaving. If it is inconclusive, the epileptologist will likely order another EEG later. Depending on the results, more EEG exams will be done before any decisions about reducing medication are made.

Neuropsychological Testing:

Depending on your cognitive and mental progress, neuropsychological testing may be done 6 months to a year after surgery. Any necessary therapy to help you get to your postoperative baseline will begin following the testing. This is a case-by-case situation, and not all patients need to have any neuropsychological testing after surgery.

There are many components that factor in to determine the normal course of events during and after epilepsy surgery. While we can offer typical expectations for this timeline, it is important to remember that your individual surgery experience may vary. It is best to openly discuss any uncertainties or questions you have with your medical team and hospital staff to know how best to prepare. In the next chapter, we discuss commonly asked questions that can serve as a guide for where to begin the discussion with your medical team.

CHAPTER EIGHT
FREQUENTLY ASKED QUESTIONS ABOUT
EPILEPSY SURGERY

As you get closer to making a decision about epilepsy surgery, you may still have many questions and concerns. In this chapter, we address patients' frequently asked questions about the procedure, the hospital stay, and long-term recovery in a systematic way. By no means will this chapter cover all possible questions and answers, but it summarizes the most common ones.

Before Surgery

What Should I Bring to the Hospital?
Bring comfortable clothes. Button-down shirts are preferable because they are easy to remove and put back on during an electroencephalogram (EEG) and when your head is wrapped after surgery. You should also bring items to help you stay occupied during the hospital stay, such as books and portable electronics such as a laptop or tablet. Parents of patients should bring their child's favorite toys, books, and games, as well as any favorite stuffed animal or toy that will make the hospital stay easier. Consult your hospital policy because it varies between centers.

Will I Have the Surgery the Same Day I Am Admitted?
Yes, you will be admitted the day of the operation. You will be called the day before to discuss what time to arrive at the hospital. All the pre-operative testing is done 1–2 weeks before the surgery day at pre-admission testing (PAT).

Will I Need a Blood Transfusion?
Most likely not. The incision for epilepsy surgery is relatively small, and blood loss is usually minimal for epilepsy surgery. However, in some cases, such as with hemispherectomies or other large operations, it may be necessary

If I Do Need a Transfusion, Can I Donate My Own Blood?
Patients or family members can donate their own blood for use during their surgery, but this varies based on hospital procedure. This is called *directed*

donor blood, and the surgical team can make these arrangements for you to do this. Patients who wish to donate their own blood must do so at least 2 weeks before surgery.

How Much of My Hair Will Be Removed?
Whether your head needs to be shaved depends on the type of surgery you are having, so you will have to ask your doctor or nurse. Sometimes little to no hair will need to be shaved; sometimes the entire head will be shaved. Surgeons may have their own preference of how much hair to shave, so it is very much a case-by-case situation. If you have long hair and only part of the hair needs to be shaved, you will be able to brush the rest of the hair over the bald spot. Some patients choose to have their entire heads shaved so an even layer of hair grows back; but again, it is a case-by-case situation.

What Type of Anesthesia Will Be Used?
Patients are put under general anesthesia and are asleep for the operation. You will meet with the anesthesiologist prior to the surgery in pre-admission testing and again on the day of the operation to talk about the type of anesthesia that will be used.

What Happens During the Time Between Grid Placement and Surgery in a Multistage Surgery?
Some people think they will be able to go home between the two procedures. However, you will remain in the hospital throughout this time.

What Is It Like to Be in the Hospital?
For some patients, the hospital can be a scary place, especially following a major procedure like epilepsy surgery. It's good to note that most people do not enjoy being in the hospital for a number of reasons, and being uncomfortable is not unusual. Pain around the incision, along with headaches, will be normal, but medication will be available to alleviate the pain. Eating and drinking normally will take a few days, as pain medications can suppress appetite. Most patients spend a lot of time sleeping or resting, which is encouraged in the immediate days after surgery. In multistage surgery, you will be on bed rest from the time the electrodes are implanted. However, you are encouraged to move around in bed, do deep breathing exercises, and move your legs. Members of the surgical team will help you with this.

Will I Need Physical Therapy?

Most patients do not need physical therapy after surgery. You receive physical therapy and occupational therapy during the hospital stay to speed up your recovery and increase endurance following surgery. Most patients do not need any additional physical therapy when they leave the hospital; but if you do, the surgical team will make arrangements.

How Long Will I Be In The Hospital?

This depends largely on the surgical plan and will be reviewed with you during the surgical consultation. Patients undergoing epilepsy surgery can be in the hospital for as little as 2–3 days to more than a month. It depends on what testing is required, the type of surgery, and the recovery time. For example, a two-stage procedure will typically require hospitalization for an average of 10–14 days, during which time there will be video-EEG monitoring, mapping, and the surgery itself. A patient having temporal lobe surgery without prior intracranial EEG, however, could be discharged home 2–3 days after surgery. It all depends on how a patient tolerates pain, how able he or she is to intake food and liquids, and the person's overall comfort level.

Who Will Be in the Operating Room (OR) During the Surgery?

It depends on the facility, but in general the surgeon, a physician's assistant, one or two scrub nurses, a circulating nurse, and an anesthesiologist will be present. In a teaching hospital, one or more neurosurgery residents will be in the OR as well.

How Expensive Is the Surgery?

It varies greatly depending on where you live. Most government plans and insurance carriers usually cover epilepsy surgery, but sometimes insurance does not cover portions of the costs. All of this will be determined before the surgery. Some surgeons do not accept medical insurance and may charge upward of $15,000 per surgical case. Some plans have co-pays and deductibles, and the cost variability is enormous. Although the surgeon's office or hospital is required to have prior authorization before the surgery, you should also check with your insurance and the hospital beforehand to know what your financial responsibility will be.

Immediately Following Surgery and Hospital Recovery

When and Where Will I Be Transferred After Surgery?
Generally, a patient goes from surgery directly to the neurosurgical intensive care unit (NSICU) or to the recovery room or post-anesthesia care unit (PACU) for a few hours. Then you will be moved to the intensive care unit (ICU) or pediatric intensive care unit (PICU) and stay there overnight. The next day, you will be transferred to the epilepsy unit for the invasive monitoring period and then to the neurology or epilepsy unit, but it depends on the facility and how you are doing. Some hospitals keep patients in ICU during the invasive monitoring study.

Can Parents or Spouses Stay Overnight in the ICU, PICU, or Recovery Room?
Yes, but it is not necessary. If they wish, parents or spouses may be able to stay in the patient's room, depending on that particular hospital's policy and based on the patient's needs.

Will I Have Staples or Stitches in My Head?
It depends on the type of surgery and the surgeon. However, it is becoming more common for surgeons to use staples. Generally, they will be removed about 10–14 days after the surgery, depending on the procedure, in an outpatient office visit.

Will There Be Any Metal Pieces in My Skull/Head After the Surgery?
There will be small titanium screws and plates in your skull that are compatible with magnetic resonance imaging (MRI) and will not set off metal detectors.

What Will the Incision Look Like?
The incision may be discomforting to look at for some people. Normally, the incision is small and unnoticeable because of the stitches or staples. It may stay pink-ish for a few months until the skin color returns to normal.

How Much Swelling Will There Be?
The swelling will appear on the side of the head with the incision. Swelling can start soon after surgery and may last several days.

Who Will Care for Me in the Hospital After Surgery?

It depends on the hospital. Usually, the neurosurgeon and his or her team will care for you after surgery. Sometimes, the ICU physician takes the lead as far as monitoring your medications and post-surgery health. In some centers, both teams will share the care responsibilities. The neurosurgeon and neurologist should communicate with each other frequently about your post-surgical care.

Can I Wear Glasses or Headphones After My Surgery?

If the legs of your glasses can be removed, the front part of your eyeglasses can be taped around the dressing. If your headphones can be adjusted, you may be able to wear them. Headphones that fit directly inside the ear are easier to wear than those that wrap around the top of the head.

What Kind of Pain Medicine Will I Be On?

Pain is very subjective, and each patient will tolerate pain differently. Most patients will receive pain drugs like morphine for a few days after surgery, after which they are transitioned onto other pain medications. Other patients may only take acetaminophen or mild pain medications. The most important point about pain control is that you should tell your doctor or nurse if you have pain or not. There is no reason to suffer in pain if it can be alleviated.

What Are the Side Effects of These Pain Medications?

Morphine and other narcotics can cause nausea, constipation, sedation, or dizziness. If you can use acetaminophen with codeine instead of stronger medicines, you may experience fewer side effects. Transitioning to milder pain medications will help to alleviate the side effects, and your surgical team will work closely with you to ensure you are kept comfortable throughout the hospitalization, during the transition at home, and through complete recovery.

Will I Be on Antibiotics?

Normally, you will only be on antibiotics during surgery and the day after surgery. It varies based on surgeon preference and hospital protocols.

Can I Get Out of Bed to Go to the Bathroom After the Surgery?

You will most likely have to use a bedpan or a bedside commode after the surgery for the first day. After that, another person can accompany you to the bathroom. If you have electrodes implanted, you will be on bed rest. You may be allowed to use a bedside commode, but it depends on the type of seizures you have, the amount of medication you're on, and on the hospital policy.

Is It Normal to Have a Few Seizures After the Surgery?

Not necessarily. In some patients, one or two breakthrough seizure may occur for no identifiable reason. Seizures are most likely to occur after surgery if you miss doses of medication, or if the medication levels in your bloodstream are low. Although the return of seizures can be psychologically devastating, having a seizure after surgery does not mean that seizure control cannot be restored. The longer the interval of seizure freedom after surgery, the greater the chances are of you never having another seizure. However, if typical seizures return on a frequent basis, there is a greater possibility that seizures may return.

Will Having Surgery Change My Personality?

Having surgery can make you feel as if you are on an emotional roller coaster. Some people will experience a surge in emotion after the surgery, sometimes feeling euphoria (extreme happiness) or a need to cry for no reason. These feelings should subside over time. Sometimes, it is possible for pre-existing personality traits to be exacerbated after surgery, but this is not very common and also tends to subside. One exception to this rule is that patients having frontal lobe resection may become more emotional, more easily distracted, or more impulsive after surgery. You should discuss the potential for these changes beforehand with your epileptologist and surgeon.

Long-Term Recovery

When Can I Go Back to Work or School?

It depends on the type of surgery, how you feel, and the type of work you do. Most people will not be able to go back to work within 4–6 weeks, although some patients may go back to work much sooner. You should not try to do too much, too soon. It is important to gradually get back into a typical work or school routine, perhaps working an hour or two a day, until you are ready to work for an entire day. You should discuss with your surgeon and epileptologist what will be best for you.

Will I Have to Wear the Head Dressing when I Leave the Hospital?

No. The large surgical bandage or head wrap will be removed before you go home, and a small dressing will be applied.

Will It Hurt When the Stitches/Staples Are Removed? Does One Hurt More Than the Other?

Generally, the skin is still numb because the nerves have not regrown yet. Most patients do not find staple removal uncomfortable and will not ask for pain medication. Removing stitches can be more uncomfortable, however, and medication will be available if you need it. Generally, patients report that they feel better once the stitches/staples have been removed.

How Long Will It Take Before I Feel Completely Normal Again?

Recovery time is variable and is very individualized. You will feel better and better gradually, and most patients report feeling completely recovered within about 6 months.

What Should I Do if I Start to Feel Depressed During Recovery or Experience a Mood Change?

Just like discomfort from pain, emotional discomfort should be discussed with your surgical team and epileptologist right away. Sometimes short-term medication may be helpful to lessen this discomfort while healing takes place.

Will Surgery Affect My Sex Drive/Libido?

This is not usually reported, but that does not mean it does not occur. Please discuss this with the surgery team if it does. It is okay to resume sexual relations a couple of weeks after surgery.

How Long Before I Can Exercise Again?

Patients are encouraged to begin walking daily right after surgery and to gradually increase the distance every few days. Working out and strenuous physical activity can resume in about 4 weeks after surgery, but it must be gradual. Please discuss the specifics of your exercise routine with your surgical team so you can get help developing an individualized plan.

Will Have Any Short- or Long-Term Memory Loss as a Result of Surgery? Is Forgetfulness Normal?

Patients often complain of short-term memory loss before the surgery as a result of uncontrolled seizures, so surgery that controls the seizures will often stop this continued memory decline. There should be no long-term memory effects following surgery.

What Else Can I Do to Treat Headaches After Surgery Besides Taking Painkillers?

Avoid stress and strenuous activities. Utilize stress-relieving therapies such as meditation, deep breathing exercises, and guided imaging. Get plenty of sleep each night (8 hours), and take extra rest and naps during the day if you feel tired. Acetaminophen (Tylenol) is often effective for controlling pain, and using an ice pack or cool towel can help. You can also use anti-inflammatory medication such as ibuprofen (Motrin or Advil) for pain management a week after surgery.

Can I Have Caffeine After Surgery and During My Recovery Period?

Yes, in moderation. However, you should not have any caffeine after 5 p.m.

What If I Have a Seizure During My Recovery at Home?

Report this to your surgical team and epileptologist right away.

How Long Will It Take Before the Doctor Can Start Reducing My Medication?

This is very individualized and based on seizure history and the type of surgery that was done. If there is no seizure activity reported during your follow-up EEG, your doctor may consider reducing your medication dose slightly in as little as 6 months after surgery. If you remain seizure-free for a certain amount of time, your doctor may continue to reduce your medication. Some patients are not mentally ready to begin weaning off their medications, however, and you should thoroughly discuss any hesitations you have with your doctor before any changes are made.

Will I Have Medication Withdrawals from Reducing Medication?

Medication reduction is done very slowly and methodically to avoid any uncomfortable side effects such as withdrawal symptoms. Generally speaking, patients feel better when they come off some of their medication. Often patients are more comfortable staying on at least one medication. The primary goals of the surgery are freedom from seizures without any surgical complications. Medication reduction is an added benefit.

How Long Will It Take for My Memory to Start to Improve If I

Become Seizure-Free After Surgery?

Continued memory decline will cease and plateau after surgery if you achieve seizure control.

Is There Anything You Can Do If the Surgery Is Not Successful?

Physicians may determine that an additional surgery to remove more brain tissue is needed. This is discussed in other chapters, and it is a complex issue. You should discuss this with your neurologist and surgeon.

Frequently Asked Questions by Parents of Children Aged 0–5

What Can We Do to Comfort Our Child While in the Hospital?
Here are some tips from other parents:

- Let your child watch his or her favorite movies, do puzzles, or play games—something that he or she enjoys that requires concentration. It will pass the time and help take his or her mind off being in the hospital.
- Create a list of fun things that you are going to do together in the hospital after the surgery so there is something to look forward to.
- Encourage siblings and extended family to visit.
- Make use of resources in the pediatric service, like child life specialists, recreation specialists, music therapists, and teachers. They can all provide additional activities and support. Depending on your child, doing schoolwork and reading may also create a sense of a normalcy and provide comfort.

What Will It Be Like for My Child Right After the Surgery?
Usually, children do very well after surgery. They may be cranky and cry for a few hours, but by the next day, most kids are back to playing and eating normally. As with adults, pain control and food intake drives the entire situation. What is different is that kids want to play, and anything that helps them in that respect will make the post-op care easier.

When Can My Child Go Back to School?
Most children can return to school in about 4–6 weeks. When possible, the child should be home-schooled during this time, so he or she does not fall too far behind the rest of his or her classmates. It is also helpful to schedule play dates with other children their age, so that the child continues to develop social skills.

CHAPTER NINE
THE PATIENT'S PERSPECTIVE:
PERSONAL STORIES

Introduction

The road to epilepsy surgery is often a winding, bumpy one of sorts. The time between diagnosis and recovery can be what feels like a lifetime for the person suffering from uncontrolled seizures. While healthcare specialists, family, and friends are invaluable support systems throughout this journey, it's not uncommon for epilepsy patients to feel alone— wondering if anyone can *truly* relate. You can consult with the most qualified doctors, read every piece of medical literature, and lean on your loved ones for guidance, but understanding and coming to terms with epilepsy surgery from a fellow patient's perspective is often the missing puzzle piece. In an endless cycle of coping with seizures, medications, medical tests, social conflicts, and disabilities, connecting with another epilepsy patient can be like finding the long-lost twin you never knew you had—finally, someone who understands the often unexplainable, uncomfortable, embarrassing, debilitating life of living with seizures.

Even more than that, a patient's perspective offers a unique insight into the unspoken struggles of life with epilepsy and the rocky path to surgery. Whatever fears, concerns, and internal conflicts you're harboring during this limbo between a life with uncontrolled seizures and a life free of them, take comfort in knowing that they have been and are shared by millions of fellow patients. There is another side to epilepsy; there is a life beyond seizures; and there is hope for a better tomorrow. Surgery is not necessarily the easiest path, but for those who are candidates, it can be the life-changing one. In these unfiltered patient accounts, we hope to provide you with answers to any final questions—both asked and unasked—as well as offer a source of comfort so that you know that you are not alone.

—Two-time epilepsy surgery patient (seizure-free for 2 years),
Foram M.

Living WITH Epilepsy

The debilitating consequences of a life with uncontrolled seizures are a universal truth all epilepsy patients know too well. Regardless of the type of seizures you suffer from or how often they occur, it's nearly impossible to quantify an epilepsy patient's suffering due to this condition. The risk of physical injuries aside, it's arguably the cognitive, emotional, and social repercussions that heavily disable the patient. Quality of life diminishes greatly as you anticipate the next unpredictable seizure while concurrently struggling with the cognitive damage and, for many patients, adverse side effects from anti-seizure medication.

Here is recent surgery patient, Sylvia,* a 24-year-old with an all too common story of life with uncontrolled seizures.

"When my doctor diagnosed me with epilepsy, I was in my final year of graduate school for occupational therapy at the time. I knew I had heard him correctly; but at the same time, I didn't want to believe it. It was a really tough year, and I was barely passing my classes because of damage I was experiencing from the frequent complex partial seizures. It inevitably took a toll on my studies.

"To make it worse, my medication was making me very dizzy. Wherever I would go, I was scared. I didn't know if I would have a seizure, or, if I had just taken my medication, if I would be able to talk to people normally. I didn't have any control, and it made me very insecure. Losing the ability to drive was also incredibly upsetting. I shouldn't have felt this way, but I often felt burdensome to my family because they had to take me everywhere I needed to go, even when it was out of their way."

Feelings of debilitation and dependency can lead many patients to feel unnecessarily remorseful, compounding the already existing emotional stress—a common byproduct of repetitive, uncontrolled seizures. However, for patients who are also heads of families, the conundrum is how to overcome the disabilities and still be able to provide for those leaning on you. Epilepsy patients are children, siblings, and friends, but they are also spouses, mothers, and fathers—people whose weighty responsibilities to care for their families do not allow them to succumb to the stress of a life with unpredictable episodes. These patients sometimes struggle with the decision of whether or not to have surgery because they know the outcome won't only affect them. For them, the risks and benefits of surgery must be weighed even more carefully.

James N., 47, shares the conflicting feelings he experienced when, after nearly a decade of living with seizures, his doctors warned him that although surgery could potentially offer him a seizure-free life, it could also result in other disabling complications.

"I underwent all the pre-surgical testing, and the doctors agreed that I was a 'good' candidate for resective surgery and that I had a high percentage probability of a seizure-free life.

"The problem was that the portion of my brain to be removed was located on the dominant side, and the doctors said it seemed to be functioning perfectly, according to the WADA test—meaning it was likely I'd suffer 'moderate to severe short-term memory loss.' Given that I was a high-functioning attorney and CPA working within an intense industry, my doctor told me that I would not likely be able to continue to function at that high of a level. I was married with kids reliant on me. So, given the risks, I deemed it 'unfair' to them that I bear a risk that could affect them so greatly.

"I continued to live with seizures and switched doctors 7 years later. I had since had three more children and reality was sinking in that my seizures had gotten worse. Although living with [the seizures] was my family's norm, it was becoming harder and scarier to live with, as the seizures had increased in frequency over the years. More people had seen me have them in my life, so I had to limit what I could do with my kids. It became more difficult to be present during business meetings and social functions with family and friends without the fear of a seizure.

"As I got older, the impact that it was not a passing thing and it was here to stay had sunk in and I was so embarrassed about it all the time. I received another opinion on my previous test results, and my new doctors helped me feel more comfortable with all my fears and concerns regarding the chance of complications. I recognized things would get worse over time if I did not have surgery, so I had no choice. My family and I had no other option."

Just as any daily occurrence quickly becomes routine, the regularity of uncontrolled seizures can significantly alter the day-to-day norm for an epilepsy patient. When your everyday events are centered on the next seizure, the slightest changes to routine must be monitored carefully. For an epilepsy patient, this sobering reality leaves very little room to "go with the flow."

Virgil B., 39, offers a snippet into the life he led for 35 years before opting for resective surgery.

> *"I had had a handful of grand mal seizures over my lifetime, but I would have countless complex partial seizures over just a couple of days. I had them so regularly that I thought it was fantastic if I went a week and didn't have one. What was worse is that something so normal as being tired would mean I'd have multiple seizures daily."*

Making the Choice for Surgery

Being offered with an opportunity to be seizure-free is like finally seeing the light at the end of the tunnel for epilepsy patients, many of whom have ceased to hope for a permanent cure. Of course, it is not always an easy choice to make. Major brain surgery can be a frightening concept for even the most courageous human being. However, when faced with the dismal reality of deteriorating brain function and a lifelong disability, brain surgery offers a very real possibility for new life. For patients fortunate enough to be candidates for surgery, opting to have the procedure can be likened to entering a lottery with multiple entries: Your chances of winning are good, but if you don't enter, there's only one end result.

Here is Richard S., 55, on how he overcame his worries about having surgery after many unsuccessful attempts to control his seizures with medication for more than a decade.

> *"My fear was whether the surgery would change who I was as a person. I thought I was going to be someone completely different if they removed a piece of my brain. It was a fear of the unknown. So when my doctor suggested the procedure, I cried to him and said 'I don't want to have brain surgery.'*
>
> *"But he told me plainly that no drug would ever control my seizures, and, over time, the memory loss, cognitive damage, and depression would eventually be what changed me. It was that moment that I realized I had to do it. You have to really ask yourself, which is worse? Everything is a choice. I made the choice to beat epilepsy*

145

with surgery, and I won."

While a fear of surgical complications or an unsuccessful outcome is very normal and readily discussed, the fear of a new life without seizures is not uncommon. For patients who have known nothing else but how to live with a disability, the possibility of being faced with new challenges—and no crutch—is equally unsettling. Worries about failure, newfound independence, and the unknown are not as easy to speak about openly. After all, who *doesn't* want to be seizure-free? But seizure freedom can be a frightening concept for someone who has known only how to live with seizures. For this reason, especially, it's important to remember that the choice to have surgery is very much an emotional one as a logical one.

Adria G., 61, remembers the internal struggle she faced when posed with an opportunity to be seizure-free after living with uncontrolled epilepsy for 25 years.

> *"I never said it out loud, but I thought to myself, do I want to give up being a handicap? Do I want to give up having this disability that allows me not to have to do certain things? And that was a big decision—it took me a long time to decide. I sat there wondering, do I really want to do this and give up my crutch?*
>
> *"Then I had a grand mal seizure while walking to my doctor's office in New York City. I fell in between two parked cars and came out of it with people helping me to get back up. When I finally made it to my doctor's office, I realized I had broken my rib and I couldn't even speak. When I came out of that seizure, I thought to myself, I give up—I'm going to have to do the surgery. I didn't know if it would cure me, I knew things would be better."*

Nearly all patients will agree that a strong support network is incredibly influential in making the choice for surgery an easier one. A medical team that is both highly skilled and makes you feel at ease is invaluable—for you and your loved ones. Your doctor, surgeon, and the rest of the surgical team should offer you comfort as well as medical care. It is perfectly okay—in fact, it is recommended—that you choose a medical team that you fully trust to provide you with the best medical and emotional support for a successful surgery and speedy recovery. Here is Sylvia sharing an experience that she says deeply impacted her comfort level and her advice to fellow patients on finding the right team.

"Before they wheeled me into the OR, I was in the waiting room with my parents. When they took me into surgery, I was so surprised when my surgeon asked where my parents were? He visibly got frustrated that they had brought me in without my parents—and that just made the world to me because he wanted to keep my parents in the loop. He wanted that for me because he knew it was a scary time for me. He was just amazing—he knew how to take care of me.

"My surgeon's entire team was wonderful. They explained everything so well and really tried to accommodate to my needs before and after the surgery. It made the entire process easier. If you don't have someone that makes you feel this comfortable, keep looking. Keep searching until you find somebody that you feel you can put your life in his or her hands."

Recovering from Surgery

Both healthcare professionals and fellow surgery patients will unanimously agree that the road to recovery is not an easy one. The first step to a successful recovery is accepting this reality and, second, setting realistic expectations. Additionally, while your healthcare team and fellow patients can help prepare you for what's "normal" during recovery, it's especially important to remember that no two cases are identical, and each patient heals at his or her own pace. As we discussed in the previous chapters, pain, fatigue, and depression are all very common during this time; however, to what degree and how long you'll experience them is case by case. For some patients, severe headaches and discomfort is the predominant struggle during recovery; for others, it is the unexpected toll on their emotional and mental well-being.

Though it's difficult to predict the standard length of recovery before you will feel "normal" again, patients should focus on the fact that it is a gradual process. By practicing good nutrition and light exercise, resting, and making an active effort to stay positive, you can expect to feel better gradually in the coming weeks and months.

Here's Virgil again, aptly describing a typical experience in the immediate weeks following a temporal lobectomy procedure and his advice for potential surgery patients.

"It was very hard to engage me in conversation in the first 2 months after surgery. I would wake up on some days and simply not want to talk to anyone. It required a lot of patience from my family and friends. I felt almost like my entire body was waking up slowly for 2 months.

"Something else I remember experiencing was having to think about things very slowly and take my time with everything. Everything from my physical coordination to my mental capacity to process thoughts and tasks was slow; I was very absent-minded. I also fatigued so easily. If I started my day in the early morning, I would feel like it was the end of the day by noon.

"You also become extremely emotional about things—I felt like a 2-year-old sometimes. You should be prepared to know that life can be very frustrating during this time. But all of this is normal.

"You have to be very, very patient and not expect too much of yourself. My surgeon told me it would take me a full year to recover, and he was telling the truth. So don't feel bad if you're not feeling 'right' after 4 months—it's a process. You will gradually start to feel better and better, and, every few months, you'll realize how much more you've recovered. At the end of the year, you'll feel like 'Wow, this is normal.'"

Though headaches and pain at the incision site are very common during recovery, not all patients report the same degrees of discomfort. Richard, whom we heard from earlier, remembers his observations while recovering from surgery. Like Virgil, Richard recalls struggling with an onset of depression and talks about dealing with it 11 years after his surgery.

"There were two surprises during recovery: One was that I couldn't chew because all the muscles on the side of my face where I was operated on were so sore. Other than that—and having a sore behind from laying in a hospital bed for days—I really didn't experience much pain.

"There was only one time at home that I felt pain, and it was very brief. I felt a very sharp pain at the incision site, which I believe was normal. But it didn't last long at all.

"The other surprise was the depression. I found myself crying without realizing it. There was never a genuine trigger for it. I had temporal lobe epilepsy, and I think I had some amount of depression even before the operation. The surgery seemed to

148

exaggerate the depression, but I didn't know to expect that. My parents pointed out once that I wouldn't get off the couch during the recovery period. I didn't think anything of it at the time, but in retrospect, I realize it was the depression.

"Though it's not to the same degree, I still experience a little bit of depression today and take antidepressants for it, but I don't have seizures any more."

A fear of returning seizures is also very common post-surgery, particularly in patients who lived many years expecting unexpected seizures. Though one can argue that there is no truly "getting used to" living with uncontrolled seizures, patients like Virgil offer a glimpse into how a life filled with sporadic seizure episodes is ironically very normal for people like him. Coming to terms with the reality that your day-to-day may no longer revolve around anticipating the next seizure is an adjustment process for all successful surgery patients. Naturally, it takes time to accept and fully believe that seizures are a thing of the past and that life can be "normal" without them. Any accompanying fear, anxiety, and nervousness during this period are only to be expected during this already emotionally taxing time— especially while you learn to live without this debilitating condition. Here is James with a relatable experience among successful surgery patients.

"I was prepared for pain and tiredness, but I was not prepared for the fear I experienced after the surgery. I became so fearful of seizures reoccurring that I had panic attacks and needed professional counseling for the first time in my life. Apparently this reaction is normal. The psychological stress improved significantly over time, but I did not ever guess or know that I would experience this during recovery. Most of the surgery patients I spoke with lived with seizures for a much shorter time than I did, so they did not seem to experience the fears that I had post-op. I had suffered seizures for more than 17 years and I learned to deal with them, so I needed more time to accept and trust that I deserved to live a seizure-free life forever."

Accepting Life After Surgery

With today's advanced technology and epilepsy knowledge, surgery candidates have every reason to be optimistic that they could one day be seizure-free. Many patients—a few mentioned here—are living proof it is possible. Though positivity and optimism are invaluable before and after surgery, it's equally as important to remember that 100 percent seizure freedom is impossible to guarantee in all patients. Should you experience a setback, working closely with your medical team and exploring your options can still allow you to live a much-improved life. Roxanne D., 43, shares her post-surgery experience and how she dealt with her seizures returning.

> *"I was excited and just ready to get the surgery over with. My daughter was a baby at the time, and I didn't want her to remember me going through the surgery. The doctors told me I had a 90 percent chance of having seizure freedom, and for 7 years I was seizure-free, but they eventually came back very sporadically because there is some remaining scar tissue. I'm a candidate to have surgery again, but I had a very difficult recovery and don't want to go through it again. I chose to have the VNS [vagus nerve stimulation] system implanted, and it's done a lot for me.*
>
> *"Stress and lack of sleep increases the likelihood I'll have a seizures, but as long as I take my medication on a timely schedule, it's okay. I am optimistic that with the right medication and settings, I could be seizure-free."*

Being fully prepared for the risk of other complications, both minor and major, is equally as important. Patients must realize and accept that there is a chance that a complication could affect your quality of life, even if only slightly. Only by thoroughly discussing the various risks with your medical team can you know the full weight of what can happen. Ultimately, focusing on the best outcome can help you make the best decision for you.

Our recent surgery patient, Sylvia, experienced a complication during her two-part resective surgery that left her with double vision. Though she faces a new challenge, Sylvia is currently seizure-free with full hope from her medical team that she will remain that way. She provides insight on how she's coming to terms with the outcome and what advice she has for anyone who fears the same.

> *"Look into yourself and ask yourself what you want from life? What do you want for yourself in the future? If seizures are in any way hindering you from getting what you want, consider surgery. It has changed my life for the better, and it can do the same for you. I have double vision…I don't feel regret. Right now, I'm accepting*

it for what it is and moving forward by doing the best that I can to live with this. I'm hopeful that, like the seizures, it'll get better over time."

Of course, patient anecdotes vary from person to person. Each patient has his or her own story to share, complete with personal struggles and victories. While no two stories are identical, connecting with fellow patients offers a one-of-a-kind insight into the epilepsy surgery experience that is unique only to those who have experienced it first-hand. If for no other reason, speaking to fellow patients provides a confirmation that you are neither the first nor the last to challenge epilepsy—but you can be the next patient to overcome it.

CHAPTER TEN
PATIENT RESOURCES

Introduction

For more information on commonly prescribed seizure medications and medical devices, patients can contact the following pharmaceutical and medical device companies:

Abbvie Pharmaceuticals (Depacon, Depakote)
- *Homepage: www.abbvie.com, www.depakote.com*
- *Contact:* 1-800-255-5162

Teva Pharmaceuticals (Gabitril)
- *Homepage: www.tevausa.com, www.gabitril.com*
- *Contact:* 1-800-896-5855

Glaxo Smith Kline (Lamictal)
- *Homepage: www.gsk.com*
- *Contact:* 888-825-5249

Novartis (Tegretol, Trileptal)
- *Homepage: www.pharma.us.novartis.com*
- *Contact:* 862-778-2100

Janssen Pharmaceuticals, Inc. (Topamax)
- *Homepage: www.janssenpharmaceuticalsinc.com, www.topamax.com*
- *Contact:* 1-800-526-7736

Pfizer (Cerebyx, Dilantin, Neurontin, Zarontin, Lyrica)
- *Homepage: www.pfizer.com, www.lyrica.com*
- *Contact:* 1-800-879-3477

Genentech (Klonopin)
- *Homepage*: *www.genentech.com*
- *Contact*: 877-436-3683

Shire (Carbatrol)
- *Homepage*: *www.shire.com*
- *Contact*: 1-888-227-3755

UCB Pharma (Keppra, Keppra XR, Vimpat)
- *Homepage*: *www.ucb-usa.com*
- *Contact*: 1-844-599-2273

Meda Pharmaceuticals (Felbatol)
- *Homepage*: *http://www.medapharma.us/*, *www.felbatol.com*
- *Contact*: 732-564-2200

Valeant Pharmaceuticals International, Inc. (Diastat, Mysoline)
- *Homepage*: *www.valeant.com*
- *Contact*: 877-361-2719

Cyberonics, Inc. (Vagus Nerve Stimulator)
- *Homepage*: *www.cyberonics.com*
- *Contact*: 800-332-1375

NeuroPace (RNS System)
- *Homepage*: *www.neuropace.com*
- *Contact*: 1-877-676-3876

Directory of Prescription Drug
Patient Assistance Programs

For prescription drug financial assistance, contact the following patient assistance programs:

AbbVie Patient Assistance Foundation (Depakote)
- *Homepage: http://www.abbviepaf.org*
- *Phone*: 1-800-222-6885
- *Address*: AbbVie Inc. 1, North Waukegan Road, North Chicago, IL 60064

Teva Cares Foundation (Gabitril)
- *Homepage: http://www.tevacares.org*
- *Phone*: 877-237-4881
- *Address*: 1090 Horsham Road, North Wales, PA 19454

GSK For You (Lamictal)
- *Homepage: www.gskforyou.com*
- *Phone*: 1-888-825-5249
- *Address*: 65 Industrial E, Clifton, NJ 07012

Patient Assistance Now (Tegretol, Tegretol XR Trileptal)
- *Homepage: www.patientassistancenow.com*
- *Phone*: 1-800-245-5356
- *Address*: P.O. Box 66556, St. Louis, MO 63166-6556

Johnson & Johnson Patient Assistance Foundation (Topamax)
- *Homepage: www.jjpaf.org*
- *Phone*: 1-800-652-6227
- *Address*: Johnson & Johnson Patient Assistance Foundation, Inc.
- Patient Assistance Program, P.O. Box 221857, Charlotte, NC 28222-1857

Pfizer RxPathways (Cerebyx, Dilantin, Neurontin, Zarontin, Lyrica)
- *Homepage*: www.pfizerrxpathways.com
- *Phone*: 877-744-5675
- *Address*: Pfizer RxPathways, P.O. Box 66976, St. Louis, MO 63166-6976

Genentech Access Solutions (Klonopin)
- *Homepage*: www.genentech-access.com
- *Phone*: 866-422-2377
- *Address*: Genentech US Drug Safety, 1 DNA Way, Mailstop 258A, South San Francisco, CA 94080

Shire Cares (Carbatrol)
- *Homepage* www.shire.com/patients/patient-services/shire-cares
- *Phone*: 1-888-227-3755
- *Address*: P.O. Box 698, Somerville, NJ 08876

UCB Patient Assistance Program (Keppra, Keppra XR, Vimpat)
- *Homepage*: www.ucb.com/patients/programmes
- *Phone*: 866-395-8366
- *Address*: UCB, Inc., P.O. Box 2198, Morrisville, PA 19067

Meda Patient Assistance Program (Felbatol)
- *Homepage*: www.felbatol.com/patient_assistance.html
- *Phone*: 866-395-8366
- *Address*: Meda Patient Assistance Program, P.O. Box 42886, Cincinnati, OH 45242

Valeant Patient Assistance Program (Diastat, Mysoline)
- *Homepage*: www.valeant.com/about/us-assistance-programs/patient-assistance
- *Phone*: 1-866-268-7325
- *Address*: P.O. Box 4008, Clinton, NJ 08809

BANZEL Patient Assistance Program (Banzel)

- *Homepage*: *www.banzel.com/banzel-patient-assistance-program.aspx*
- *Phone*: 1-888-796-1234
- *Address*: 100 Tice Blvd., Woodcliff Lake, NJ 07677

Websites

For more information on epilepsy, treatments, research, and other resources, patients can visit the following websites:

- **Epilepsy Foundation:** *www.epilepsy.com*
- **American Epilepsy Society:** *https://www.aesnet.org*
- **FACES (Finding a Cure for Epilepsy and Seizures):** *www.aces.med.nyu.edu/*
- **Advancing Epilepsy Care:** *http://www.advancingepilepsycare.com*
- **National Institute of Neurological Disorders and Stroke:** *www.ninds.nih.gov/disorders/epilepsy/detail_epilepsy.htm*

Books

For additional information on epilepsy and seizure therapies, patients' anecdotes, and resources for families of patients, the following books are available through popular book distributors. These can be found on Amazon.com:

EPILEPSY 101: The Ultimate Guide for Patients and Families, by the National Epilepsy Educational Alliance & Dr. Ruben Kuzniecky (Editor)

This patient and family guide to seizures and epilepsy was written by the leading epilepsy experts in the United States. This effort resulted in a balanced, comprehensive, and informative guide intended to inform and guide patients and families through the diagnosis, treatment, and outcome of the disorder. The text is also meant to be used as a companion helping patients with side effects, treatment options, resources, and more

Epilepsy: Patient and Family Guide, 3rd Edition, by Orrin Devinsky MD (Author)

This book offers a comprehensive and authoritative discussion of epilepsy for the patient. Written by a leading expert in the field, this extensively updated third edition incorporates many comments and suggestions from real patients and their families. This guide will answer commonly asked questions about epilepsy, dispel uncertainties and fears, and encourage those diagnosed with epilepsy to become strong advocates in their medical care. Ideal for patients or parents of children with epilepsy, this book discusses:

- The nature and diversity of seizures
- The factors that can cause or prevent seizures
- The most current information about all antiepileptic drugs
- Medical, surgical, and alternative therapies for seizures
- Legal, financial, and employment issues

Silently Seizing: Common, Unrecognized, and Frequently Missed Seizures and Their Potentially Damaging Impact on Individuals with Autism Spectrum Disorders, by Caren Haines & RN (Authors)

Up to 50% of all children diagnosed with autism have undiagnosed seizure disorders, to a great extent because they are difficult to diagnose and due to a lack of awareness and understanding. Caren Haines, with renowned behavioral child neurologist Nancy Minshew, MD, is determined to change that. At age 2, author Caren Haines's son was diagnosed with autism. By the time he was 12, his diagnosis didn't account for his uncontrollable aggression, the acrid smells that lingered in his mind, and the odd voices that screamed at him from inside his head. By the time he was 18, his out-of-control behavior mirrored a mood disorder with psychotic features. *Silently Seizing* begins with a close-up look at this family's journey and examines a disorder that cannot always be identified in a clinical setting. Intersecting at two medical subspecialties, neurology and psychiatry, the child who has autism and partial seizures is at a serious disadvantage. By inadvertently allowing children's brains to "silently seize," we are robbing children of their ability to function normally. When treated early with anti-seizure medications, many children show amazing gains in expressive language and comprehension. Many begin to speak and learn as many troubling behaviors begin to disappear. Even more important, many children lose their diagnosis of autism. Backed by up-to-the-minute research, this must-read book includes sections on what autism is, the seizure–autism connection, and tips for diagnosing and treating seizures, as well as how to better understand children's behavior.

Epilepsy: The Ultimate Teen Guide (It Happened to Me), by Kathlyn Gay & Sean McGarrahan (Authors)

Teens can lead normal, active lives despite having epilepsy, and this book shows them how other teens are doing so. Through their stories, they offer advice on whether and how to tell friends, dates, teachers, or an employer about the condition. Important teen issues, such as driving, dating, sports, and college are addressed. How the Americans with Disabilities Act (ADA) applies to people with epilepsy is also reviewed.

Let's Learn with Teddy About Epilepsy, by Dr. Yvonne Zelenka (Author) & Melissa Leyton (Illustrator)

This book is intended to help kids and families understand seizures and epilepsy using an illustrated story about a young boy, his best friend, and his family. Teddy has a seizure for the first time in his life. The book goes through the symptoms, the diagnosis, tests, and treatment. The book is intended to help children cope with the disorder and understand the tests and treatment. The story ends with a powerful message in that Teddy is not in any way different from the boy he was prior to the seizure.

I Have Epilepsy. It Doesn't Have Me, by Jamie Bacigalupo, Judy Bacigalupo (Authors), & Inga Shalvashvili (Illustrator)

This book follows 8-year-old Jamie on her journey from being diagnosed with benign rolandic epilepsy at age five. Jamie persevered and overcame her epilepsy and went on to help other children by starting her own nonprofit that provides gifts to children in more than five states. Proceeds go to her nonprofit to deliver to more children with epilepsy and/or asthma.

Mommy, I Feel Funny! A Child's Experience with Epilepsy, **by Danielle M. Rocheford (Author) & Chris Herrick (Illustrator)**
Based on a true story, this book introduces the reader to Nel, a little girl who is diagnosed with epilepsy. The story takes you through the days following Nel's first seizure. Suddenly, Nel and her family are faced with thoughts, fears, and emotions that come with the discovery, understanding, and acceptance of epilepsy.

Epilepsy Unveiled: Caretaking, Seizures, Psychosis and Brain Surgery, **by Lola Jines-Burritt (Author)**
Are you blindly stumbling down unfamiliar paths created by living with epilepsy? Are you looking for answers as the caretaker of someone who has seizures? Is your world abnormal due to seizures? Are you witnessing irrational behaviors and unable to find an answer to them? Are you living behind closed doors and smothered by misunderstanding? Have you decided your fate is sealed and stopped looking for answers? Lola Jines-Burritt and her husband Charley began their journey with his epilepsy in 1980 and observed every imaginable aspect of epilepsy for 26 years. The goal of her book is to educate others, both those with epilepsy from various causes and their caretakers. The book focuses on the link between epilepsy and psychosis. This book also contains information to help with recognizing different seizure types and responding to them, being a competent caretaker while sheltering the one you love, finding balance between being protective and promoting individuality for the person who has seizures, adjusting to epilepsy as a caretaker and a person who suffers with seizures, managing the public and medical community, identifying clusters of seizures and understanding psychosis, paralleling medical terms with recognizable psychotic behaviors, comprehending delusions and identifying hallucinations, preparing for all aspects of brain surgery including the steps before and adjustments afterward.

Epilepsy (What Do I Do Now), by Carl W. Bazil, Derek J. Chong, & Daniel Friedman (Authors)

Patients with epilepsy pose many clinical challenges. Even experienced clinicians occasionally arrive at the point where diagnostic, work-up, treatment, or prognostic thinking becomes blocked. Epilepsy is the fifth volume in the "What Do I Do Now" series and provides the clinician with the necessary tools to evaluate and treat an epilepsy patient. Applying a case-based approach of curbside consultation, the authors present 31 actual cases, providing key points to remember and recommendations for further reading at the end of each case and including electroencephalograms and imaging where applicable. Concise and readable, this is the perfect quick-reference guide for anyone working with epilepsy patients.

Alternative Therapies in Epilepsy Care, by Orrin Devinsky MD, Steven C. Schachter, Steven V. Pacia MD (Authors)

This book begins with an overview of the therapies themselves, including herbal remedies, nutrition, alternative pharmacological therapies, physical treatments, and neurobehavioral approaches, and also discusses medication-related considerations and caveats. The next group of chapters covers complementary and alternative medicine (CAM) and preventive approaches to mitigating the effects of epilepsy and epilepsy therapies, such as drug toxicity and the side effects of anti-epileptic drugs (AEDs), seizures, enhancing cognitive function, issues for women (pregnancy, breastfeeding, menopause), and managing anxiety and depression. The final part of the book focuses on quality of life and lifestyle modifications to reduce seizure risk, including techniques for stress reduction, sleep disturbances, alcohol and recreational drugs, and environmental factors.

Hospital Checklists

Personal Preparations to Make Prior to Surgery

❑ Inform supervisors at work/school of the surgery date and how much time I'm expected to be away.

❑ Designate a person who is in charge of communicating any changes to my expected return date to work/school should there be any.

❑ Designate a person who is in charge of keeping nonimmediate family and friends updated with news during and following the surgery.

❑ Take care of any other miscellaneous arrangements before surgery, such as paying bills or rent.

❑ Make financial arrangements for medical bills and confirm that my insurance company has cleared the surgery.

❑ Take care of any legal matters: this should include power of attorney, financial arrangements, and, last, a living will.

❑ Inform family and friends about when and where they can come to visit during the hospital stay.

❑ Inform any other people I see in my daily life (i.e., roommates, neighbors, coworkers, friends) about my surgery, so they don't worry when I'm gone and/or return from the hospital.

❑ Address any last-minute anxiety about surgery with the medical team, a therapist, or family and friends.

Final Preparations Before Surgery

- ❑ Make sure my hospital bag has the following: toiletries, warm pajamas and/or bathrobe, glasses and/or contact lenses with case, and medication for the morning.
- ❑ Make sure someone is in charge of relaying surgery updates/other information to other family and friends.
- ❑ Confirm how I'm getting to the hospital in the morning.

INDEX

Note: Boldface numbers indicate illustrations and tables.

Made in the USA
San Bernardino, CA
01 February 2017